OXFORD MEDICAL PUBLICATIONS

ANKYLOSING SPONDYLITIS

the**facts**

D1500231

the**facts**

ALSO AVAILABLE IN THE SERIES

ALCOHOLISM: THE FACTS
(third edition) Donald W. Goodwin

AUTISM: THE FACTS
Simon Baron-Cohen and Patrick Bolton

BACK AND NECK PAIN: THE
FACTS
Loïc Burn

CANCER: THE FACTS
(second edition) Michael Whitehouse
and Maurice Slevin

CHILDHOOD LEUKAEMIA: THE
FACTS
(second edition) John S. Lilleyman

CHRONIC FATIGUE SYNDROME
(CFS/ME): THE FACTS
Frankie Campling and Michael Sharpe

CYSTIC FIBROSIS: THE FACTS
(third edition) Ann Harris and Maurice
Super

DOWN SYNDROME: THE FACTS
Mark Selikowitz

EATING DISORDERS: THE FACTS
(third edition) Suzanne Abraham and
Derek Llewellyn-Jones

ECZEMA IN CHILDHOOD: THE
FACTS
David J. Atherton

EPILEPSY: THE FACTS
(second edition) Anthony Hopkins and
Richard Appleton

HEAD INJURY: THE FACTS
(second edition) Dorothy Gronwall,
Philip Wrightson and Peter Waddell

HUNTINGDON'S DISEASE: THE
FACTS
Oliver Quarrell

KIDNEY FAILURE: THE FACTS
Stewart Cameron

LUPUS: THE FACTS
Graham Hughes

MISCARRIAGE: THE FACTS
(second edition) Gillian C. L. Lachelin

MULTIPLE SCLEROSIS: THE FACTS
(fourth edition) Bryan Matthews and
Margaret Rice-Oxley

MUSCULAR DYSTROPHY: THE
FACTS
(second edition) Alan E. H. Emery

OBSESSIVE-COMPULSIVE
DISORDER: THE FACTS
(second edition) Padmal de Silva and
Stanley Rachman

PANIC DISORDER: THE FACTS
Stanley Rachman and Padmal de Silva

SCHIZOPHRENIA: THE FACTS
(second edition) Ming T. Tsuang and
Stephen V. Faraone

THYROID DISEASE: THE FACTS
(third edition) R. I. S. Bayliss and
W. M. G. Tunbridge

TOURETTE SYNDROME: THE
FACTS
(second edition) Mary Robertson and
Simon Baron-Cohen

ALSO FROM OXFORD
UNIVERSITY PRESS

FORBIDDEN DRUGS:
UNDERSTANDING DRUGS AND
WHY PEOPLE TAKE THEM
(second edition) Philip Robson

A BLOKE'S DIAGNOSE IT
YOURSELF GUIDE TO HEALTH
Keith Hopcroft and Alistair Moulds

ANKYLOSING SPONDYLITIS

the**facts**

Muhammad Asim Khan MD FACP FRCP

Professor of Medicine
Case Western Reserve University
School of Medicine, Cleveland, Ohio, USA

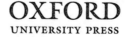

OXFORD
UNIVERSITY PRESS

OXFORD

UNIVERSITY PRESS

Great Clarendon Street, Oxford, OX2 6DP

Oxford University Press is a department of the University of Oxford.
It furthers the university's objective of excellence in research,
scholarship, and education by publishing worldwide in

Oxford New York

Auckland Cape Town Dar es Salaam Hong Kong Karachi Kuala Lumpur
Madrid Melbourne Mexico City Nairobi New Delhi Shanghai
Taipei Toronto

With offices in

Argentina Austria Brazil Chile Czech Republic France Greece
Guatemala Hungary Italy Japan South Korea Poland Portugal
Singapore Switzerland Thailand Turkey Ukraine Vietnam

Oxford is a registered trade mark of Oxford University Press
in the UK and in certain other countries

Published in the United States
by Oxford University Press Inc., New York

© Muhammad Asim Khan, 2002

A catalogue record for this title is available from the British Library

Library of Congress Cataloging in Publication Data
(Data available)

ISBN–13: 978–0–19–263282–1
ISBN–10: 0–19–263282–5

5

Printed in Great Britain
on acid-free paper by
Clays Ltd, St Ives plc

Dedication

I dedicate this book to my family (my parents, Umar and Hameeda, my wife, Mastoora, and my sons Ali and Raza), and above all to all the people like me who suffer from ankylosing spondylitis, and to their families, as well as to their healthcare providers.

Preface

This book is primarily intended for people with ankylosing spondylitis (AS), their family members and friends. I hope it will also prove useful to healthcare professionals and organizations working with AS patients.

As an academic doctor, a rheumatologist, my research interest has focused on AS and related diseases called spondyloarthropathies, which are also covered in this book. I have a more personal interest than most researchers, because I have suffered from a very severe form of AS since I was 12 years old. Some of the problems I have faced because of this disease are highlighted in two recent articles (Khan, 2000, 2001).

Early diagnosis and proper medical management of AS and related diseases can help alleviate symptoms, prevent wrong treatment, enhance the future quality of life, and help reduce the risk of long-term disability and deformity.

People with AS need to receive appropriate counseling, and also information about self-help issues, any potential lifestyle modification, and health education for enhancement of self-management. This helps them to achieve sustained health benefits while reducing healthcare costs and facilitating compliance with the recommended drug therapy and exercise regimen.

Patients who are knowledgeable about their disease have more self-responsibility, comply better with the recommended treatment regimen, and are more likely to make positive behavioral changes that will help them achieve an improved health status and outcome in the long run. This book is intended to add to their knowledge, and I hope that it will serve its intended purpose.

I am grateful to many AS self-help groups and organizations for their helpful suggestions, and in particular to Ernst Feldtkeller.

Muhammad Asim Khan MD FACP FRCP

Professor of Medicine, Case Western Reserve University School of Medicine, MetroHealth Medical Center, Cleveland, Ohio 44109, USA

Acknowledgements

I am grateful to Deutsche Vereinigung Morbus Bechterew, the German AS society, and to the National Ankylosing Spondylitis Society, the British AS societies, for permission to reproduce some figures from their publications.

- Figure 5 is reprinted with kind permission from *Atlas of rheumatology*, edited by Gene Hunder, Current Science, Philadelphia, 1998.

- Figure 7 is reprinted with kind permission from *Straight talk on spondylitis*, published by the Spondylitis Association of America.

- Figures 8–13 are reprinted with kind permission from *A positive response to ankylosing Spondylitis—a guidebook for patients*, produced by the Royal National Hospital for Rheumatic Diseases, Bath, 1998.

- Figure 14 is reprinted with kind permission from *Morbus Bechterew—ein Leitfaden für Patienten*, by Ernst Feldtkeller, Deutsche Vereinigung Morbus Bechterew (DVMB), Schweinfurt, 1985.

- Figures 15 and 20 are reprinted with kind permission from *Morbus Bechterew—ein Leitfaden für Patienten*, by Ernst Feldtkeller, Novartis Pharma Verlag, Nürnberg, 1997.

- Figure 16 is from *Bechterew-Brief*, the newsletter of DVMB, No. 78 (September 1999), p. 15. © Deutsche Vereinigung Morbus Bechterew, Schweinfurt.

- Figure 17 is from *Bechterew-Brief*, the newsletter of DVMB, No. 56 (March 1994), p. 13–16 and from *Morbus Bechterew—ein Leitfaden für Patienten*, by Ernst Feldtkeller, Novartis Pharma Verlag, Nürnberg 1997. © Detlef Becker-Capeller (Cuxhaven), schematic drawing by Ernst Feldtkeller (München), adapted from a similar drawing by Andrzej Seyfried in *Pathologische Grundlagen der Bewegungstherapie chronisch entzündlicher Gelenk- und Wirbelsäulenerkrankungen*, EULAR-Verlag Basel.

- Figure 19 is from *Primer on the rheumatic diseases*, edited by J. H. Klippel, Edition 11, page 191, Arthritis Foundation, Atlanta, Georgia, 1997.

the**facts**

CONTENTS

1	Facts and myths about ankylosing spondylitis	1
2	What is ankylosing spondylitis?	5
3	Early symptoms	13
4	The course of the disease	19
5	Exercise and physical therapy	23
6	Drug therapy	37
7	Nontraditional (complementary, or alternative) therapy	51
8	Surgical treatment	61
9	Some later manifestations	65
10	A typical case history	71
11	Living with ankylosing spondylitis: some hints	75
12	The management of AS: an overview	87
13	The rheumatologist's role	91
14	Radiology and diagnosis	95
15	The disease process	101
16	HLA-B27 and the cause of ankylosing spondylitis	111

Contents

17 Spondyloarthropathies   **125**

Appendix 1   **Ankylosing spondylitis organizations**   **143**

Appendix 2   **Glossary**   **151**
    References and further reading   **173**

Index   **183**

1
Facts and myths about ankylosing spondylitis

Facts

- Ankylosing spondylitis (or AS for short) is a chronic, progressive, painful inflammatory rheumatic disease, which affects the spinal joints, in particular those at the base of the spine (the sacroiliac joints and the lumbar spine).
- AS typically affects young people, beginning between the ages of 15 and 30. The average age of onset of the disease is 24 years, but it may range from 8 to 45 years.
- AS usually starts with chronic low back pain and stiffness which is gradual and insidious in onset. It can take a long time, on average about 6 years, before the correct diagnosis is made.
- Over many years, AS can result in gradually pro-gressive stiffness and limitations of spinal mobil-ity and also restricted expansion of the chest.
- In some people AS can affect other joints besides the spine, in particular the hip and shoulder joints. Involvement of these and other limb joints is more common in some developing countries, especially when the disease starts in childhood.

- About one-third of AS patients have one or more episodes of acute eye inflammation (acute iritis).
- AS has a characteristic appearance on X-rays, especially changes that result from inflammation of the sacroiliac joints of the pelvis (sacroiliitis). Unfortunately, this X-ray evidence may take some time to appear. An X-ray taken in the early years of the disease may be negative or indefinite (equivocal), but eventually the sacroiliac joints will show evidence of sacroiliitis.
- The disease sometimes occurs in more than one member of a family.
- The cause of AS is not yet fully known, but there is an important genetic element; most people with AS have a gene called HLA-B27. In people with AS this gene is found in over 90% of northern Europeans, about 80% of Mediterranean people, and about 50% of African-Americans. In people without AS this gene is present in only 8% of whites in the US and 2–3% of African-Americans.
- Many genes are involved, not just HLA-B27. The search is now on for these additional genes and also for the trigger factor (possibly a bacterial infection) that starts the disease processes.
- Some AS patients may also have associated psoriasis, chronic inflammatory bowel disease (ulcerative colitis and Crohn's disease) or reactive arthritis (Reiter's syndrome).
- There is no cure for AS yet, but the symptoms of back pain and stiffness usually respond well to non-steroidal anti-inflammatory drugs (NSAIDs) and a regular program of physical exercise.

- Although the course of AS is quite variable, most people with the disease do well and continue to live normal and productive lives although they may have to modify their lifestyle or their work environment. For example, a manual worker doing frequent or prolonged bending and heavy lifting may have to consider a change of job.

Myths

Myth AS is rare.

Fact AS affects at least 1 in 200 adults (approximately 0.5%), but its prevalence seems to differ in various parts of the world. A study in Germany has shown that AS affects 1% of the adult population there, making it as common as rheumatoid arthritis. AS is far more common than better-known diseases such as leukemia, muscular dystrophy, or cystic fibrosis.

Myth AS does not affect women or children.

Fact Recent studies suggest that AS is 2 to 3 times as frequent in men as it is in women. The disease may also progress more slowly in women. It can affect children, although be the disease may appear initially to be slightly different. Rather than back pain and stiffness, a child may have painful heels, knees, or hips.

Myth AS is a progressive disease that always results in a fused spine.

Fact The symptoms and severity of AS vary from one person to another. Many people do not progress to complete bony fusion of the whole spine, because the inflammation may ease off before this can happen. For people with the progressive form of AS, the inflammation does tend to spread over the years to involve the whole spine. But, although the spine becomes more stiff or rigid, the pain in the joints of the back regresses, as inflammation is replaced by a healing process that involves new bone formation. This is sometimes referred to as **burning out** of the disease. However, some occasional features of AS, such as eye inflammation (acute iritis) and heel pain, may continue to occur, suggesting that the disease may not have gone into complete remission.

Myth Nothing can be done to help the AS patient.

Fact Early diagnosis can prevent wrong treatment and help set up proper medical management that can minimize symptoms and help reduce the risk of disability and deformity.

Myth There has been no new major breakthrough in the treatment of AS patients who have failed to respond adequately to the conventional therapy.

Fact Some recent studies have shown that such patients seem to respond very well to anti-TNF therapy.

2 What is ankylosing spondylitis?

Ankylosing spondylitis (AS) is a chronic (progressive) painful inflammatory rheumatic disease that involves the back, i.e. the spine and sacroiliac joints (Figure 1). The disease typically begins in adolescence and young adulthood, and only rarely does it begin after the age of 45 years.

- The word **ankylosing** comes from the Greek root *ankylos*, meaning bent, although it has now come to imply something that restricts motion (stiffening) and may ultimately result in fusion. When the joint loses its mobility and becomes stiff it is said to be **ankylosed.**

- **Spondylitis** means inflammation of the spinal vertebrae; the word is derived from *spondylos*, which is the Greek word for vertebra, and -itis, which means inflammation. The name therefore suggests that AS is an inflammatory disease of the spine that can lead to stiffening of the back. It is sometimes called just spondylitis for short, but this word should not be confused with **spondylosis**, which relates to wear and tear in the spinal column as we get older.

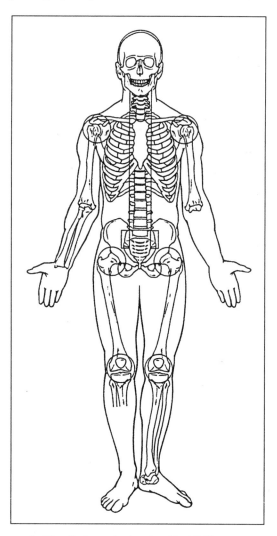

Figure 1 Sites that may be involved in AS. The most commonly involved sites are the sacroiliac joints and the spine. They are marked by rectangles. Other, relatively less commonly involved sites are hip and shoulder joints, and less often the knee joints. These sites are marked by circles.

AS in history and literature

AS has affected people since ancient times. One such sufferer was the famous Egyptian Pharaoh Ramses II. The first definite description of AS can be credited to an Irish physician, Bernard Conner (1666–1698). When he was studying medicine in France, some farmers brought him a skeleton they had found in a cemetery. He wrote that the bones were 'so straightly and intimately joined, their ligaments perfectly bony, and their articulations so effaced, that they really made but one uniform continuous bone' (Figure 2).

The first clinical descriptions of the disease date from the late nineteenth century, and the medical interest in AS was stimulated by a series of publications in the 1890s by Vladimir von Bechterew (1857–1927) in St Petersburg, Russia. Other clinical reports on AS were published by Adolf Strümpell (1853–1926) and Pierre Marie (1853–1940). Valentini published the earliest X-ray examination of a patient with AS in 1899, and in 1934 Krebs described the characteristic obliteration of the sacroiliac joints.

Although AS is a readily observed disorder in people with advanced disease, it has rarely appeared in literature. Eudora Welty mentioned it in a short story 'The Petrified Man', published in the *Southern Review* of 1938–1939.

Terminology

Over the years AS has been known by many different names, including:
• spondylitis ankylosans

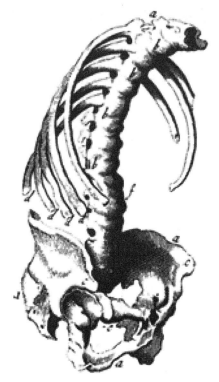

Figure 2 First representation of a skeleton with AS in its final state by Bernard Conner, London, 1695.

- spondylarthritis ankylopoetica
- morbus Bechterew (Bechterew's disease)
- morbus Strümpell–Marie–Bechterew
- Marie–Strümpell's spondylitis
- poker back.

During the first half of the twentieth century AS was wrongly called 'rheumatoid spondylitis', particularly in the USA, because of the mistaken belief that it was just a variant of rheumatoid arthritis.

Structure of the spine

The spine consists of 24 vertebrae that are stacked one above the other and held together by strong ligaments and by more than 100 joints (Figure 3). It is divided into three main sections:

- the upper part, in the neck (cervical spine) has 7 vertebrae
- the middle part (thoracic spine) has 12 vertebrae
- the lower part (lumbar spine) has 5 vertebrae.

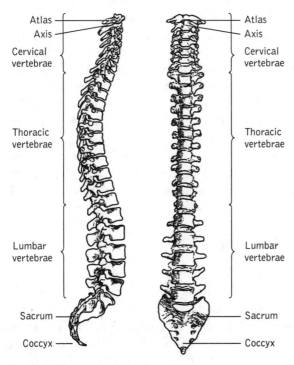

Figure 3 The vertebral column.

Each of these sections has its own gentle curvature, and the neck is the most mobile part of the spine. The 12 ribs on either side that make up the chest wall are attached to the thoracic vertebrae in the back by joints called costovertebral and costo-transverse joints, and are attached to the breastbone (sternum) in the front chest wall by costochondral junctions.

What is the sacroiliac joint?

The lowest (i.e. fifth) vertebra in the lumbar spine sits on a bone that forms the back of the pelvis. This bone is called the **sacrum**, and it looks like a keystone in the circular pelvis. It is attached on either side to the pelvic bone called the **ilium** by joints called sacroiliac joints, and by strong liga-ments (Figure 4). The front part of the pelvic bone (not shown in Figure 4) is called the pubis, and the pubic bones of the two sides form a junction in the middle called the pubic junction (or pubic sym-physis). The lower part of the pelvic bone that bears our weight when we are sitting down is called the gluteal tuberosity; there is one on either side, cush-ioned by the buttock.

Family history

AS does tend to run in families, and studies indi-cate that there is a genetic predisposition to it. This was clearly established in 1973, when researchers found a remarkable association of AS with a genetic marker called HLA-B27, which is discussed in more detail later in the book (Chapter 16). HLA-B27 is

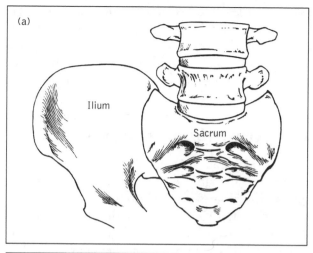

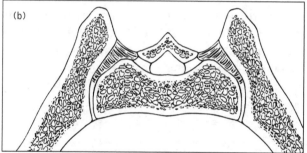

Figure 4 The sacroiliac joint: (a) location of the right sacroiliac joint marked by the line separating sacrum from ilium; (b) horizontal cross-section across both right and left sacroiliac joints—the lower part is facing the front.

found in 8% of the general white population of the USA, but in more than 90% of people with AS. The prevalence of this gene is very different in other racial groups, as also discussed in Chapter 16.

Inheriting the HLA-B27 gene does not in itself mean that you will get AS; it simply increases the probability. Current research is focusing on identification of the additional genes that pre-dispose people to AS, and the activating agent or infection that triggers the disease.

Developments in treatment

The first major advance in drug therapy in AS came with the availability of the first non-aspirin non-steroidal anti-inflammatory drugs (NSAIDs), especially phenylbutazone, in the mid-twentieth century. Many other NSAIDs have since been discovered that are safer than phenylbutazone, but none of them is more effective in relieving the pain and inflammation of AS. The latest potential break-through is the remarkable efficacy of anti-TNF therapy in AS patients who do not respond ade-quately to NSAIDs and other conventional medica-tion (see Chapter 6).

3 Early symptoms

The hallmark symptom of AS is **sacroiliitis**, the inflammation of the sacroiliac joints. The pain caused by sacroiliitis is usually a dull ache that is diffuse, rather than localized, and is felt deep in the buttock area. At first it may be intermittent or on one side only, or alternate between sides; however, within a few months it generally becomes persistent (chronic) and is felt on both sides (bilateral). Gradually the lower back becomes stiff and painful, as the inflammation extends to the spine in that area (lumbar spine). Over many months or years the back pain can gradually extend further up the spine to the area between the shoulder blades or even to the neck. These initial symptoms usually start in late adolescence or early adulthood.

Most people with AS first seek medical help when the back pain and stiffness become persistent and troublesome. Their characteristic symptoms are chronic low back pain and stiffness that have come on gradually, for no apparent reason.

The course of the disease is very variable. Some people with AS have only transient episodes of back pain with periods in between (remissions) when there are hardly any problems; others have more chronic back pain that leads to varying degrees of spinal stiffness and gradually decreasing spinal mobility. However, the spine will not always fuse completely: in some people the disease may stay limited to the sacroiliac joints and the lumbar spine.

The disease may sometimes be associated with inflammation of hip or shoulder joints (called the **girdle** joints), or the more peripheral limb joints, such as knees, ankles, or elbows. In fact, for some people, the first symptoms may not be back pain but painful girdle or limb joints. AS can be difficult to distinguish from some other rheumatic diseases when there is no back pain present. However, the typical back symptoms patients generally develop later.

Your first visit to the doctor may concern inflammation at some other sites, which then turns out to be associated with AS. For example, you may have one or more episodes of acute inflammation of the eye (acute iritis) or of the bowel (inflammatory bowel diseases such as Crohn's disease and ulcerative colitis). Many people with AS can have bowel inflammation, without being aware of any intestinal symptoms. These aspects are discussed in more detail in Chapter 15.

Pointers to early diagnosis

Back pain in the general population is very common, probably only second to the common cold as a cause of discomfort and incapacity prompting a visit to the doctor. It is the most frequent reason for temporary disability for persons under 45 years of age, and up to 80% of Americans will have a lower back problem of some type at least once by age 50.

Most people with this so-called 'nonspecific' back pain recover within 6 months, regardless of any medical care or intervention. It is only in a small proportion of people with such back pain that AS and related spondyloarthropathies are the underlying cause.

Most cases of AS can be diagnosed, or at least initially suspected, on the basis of a good medical history and a thorough clinical examination. Nevertheless, there are sometimes delays and failures in diagnosis. Your doctor can help to prevent delay in diagnosis, by distinguishing back pain due to AS from other common causes of back pain.

The back pain of early AS is usually a dull ache that is difficult to localize, felt deep in the buttock or lower back. The back pain and stiffness may be associated with muscle spasms and tenderness in the back. The symptoms are typically worse on waking up in the morning ('morning stiffness') because a long period of inactivity usually makes the pain and stiffness worse. It may even be bad enough to wake you up at night sometimes. You find it necessary to exercise or move about for a few minutes before going back to bed, and may have considerable difficulty in getting out of bed in the morning. Physical activity or a hot shower helps minimize the back pain and stiffness, and exposure to cold or dampness may make the symptoms worse. Occasionally, too, people may complain that they get fatigued easily.

For some people the back symptoms may be absent or very mild, and some may complain only of back stiffness, fleeting muscle aches, or tender areas along the back and pelvis. The problem may occasionally be misdiagnosed as 'fibrositis' or '**fibromyalgia**'.

In a thorough physical examination, the doctor should look for the presence of sacroiliitis (by noting any tenderness elicited by direct firm pressure, or pain caused by putting physical stress on the sacroiliac joints), and measure spinal mobility in all directions, including the mobility of your neck (Figure 5).

The doctor should also check for any restriction of chest expansion and examine your limbs for any signs of joint inflammation and restricted range of motion, especially of the hip and shoulder joints which are affected in one-third of patients. The limbs and the trunk, including the whole spine, the breastbone and adjacent ribs, and the heels, should be checked for any tenderness.

The ability to bend the spine backwards and sideways (without bending the knees), or to rotate the spine, is generally the first to be impaired. Many people with early AS can bend forward quite well, and even touch the ground with their fingertips, because they have good mobility in their hip joints. However, a careful examination of lumbar spinal motion using the Schober test (Figure 5g) will often detect a decrease in the forward bending flexibility of this part of their spine.

The diagnosis of AS also involves X-rays and tests to exclude other possible causes of symptoms. These are described in more detail in Chapter 14.

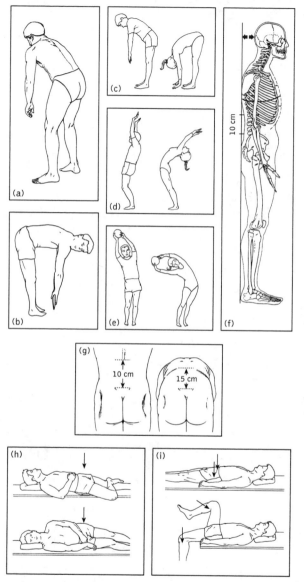

Figure 5

4
The course of the disease

AS does not follow the same course in everyone: even among affected members of one family the outcome is not exactly the same. In very early stages the symptoms may come and go, but in most people they ultimately become more persistent. However, the lower back pain and stiffness does settle down in the end, but by that time the upper part of your back and the neck may have become painful and stiff as well. It is therefore very important to maintain a good posture and prevent a stooped (bent) spine. Modern treatment can help, provided the diagnosis is made early and you comply with the recommended treatment. Most of the loss of function occurs during the first 10 years, and is correlated with the occurrence of peripheral arthritis (including hip and shoulder joints) and development of **bamboo spine**. The disease process of AS is discussed in detail in Chapter 15.

Although most of the symptoms of AS begin in the lumbar and sacroiliac areas, they may sometimes mostly involve the neck and upper back, or present as arthritis in the shoulders, hips, and feet. A variety of other problems may precede back pain and stiffness in some patients, e.g. eye inflammation (acute iritis) (see Chapter 15). Eye specialists (ophthalmologists) should always look for the possibility of underlying AS and related diseases in someone with this kind of inflammation. Restricted spinal mobility and decreased chest expansion without an obvious cause such as emphysema or scoliosis should also alert the doctor to the possibility of AS.

AS in men and women

Until a few years ago, AS was thought to be much more common in men than in women. We now know that women frequently develop the disease too, but some of them have a very mild form of the disease which may not be as easily detected as it is in men. AS has been under-diagnosed in women in the past. For example, in Germany only 10% of the AS patients diagnosed around 1960 were women, but this percentage has progressively increased since then to reach 46% among those diagnosed since 1990.

There is also a significantly longer delay in disease diagnosis for female patients, but fortunately this delay is decreasing. For example, in Germany in the 1950s there was, on average, a 15 years delay in diagnosis for women, but by 1975–79 it was down to $7\frac{1}{2}$ years.

The average age at onset of AS does not differ significantly for men and women, but the spine fusion (ankylosis) may progress more slowly in women than in men. In some women, neck and peripheral joint involvement may be the main manifestation, and some may have symptoms that resemble fibrositis (fibromyalgia) or early rheumatoid arthritis. Functional outcome, as analyzed by studying activities of daily living, is similar in men and women. However, when it comes to pain and the need for drug therapy, women with AS tend to be worse off than men. The slower and relatively incomplete progression of spinal fusion in women may mean that it takes longer for pain to decrease as a result of complete spinal ankylosis.

AS in older people

It is very rare for AS to begin after the age of 45. However, there are many people with AS whose disease is diagnosed in old age, perhaps because they have had minimal symptoms over the years. Sometimes their back pain may be due to osteoporosis or related fractures rather than to inflammation. Osteoporosis and AS in older people are discussed in detail in Chapter 9.

AS in childhood

For AS starting in childhood, i.e. up to 16 years of age (juvenile AS), knee problems may occasionally be the initial reason for consulting the doctor. Sometimes arthritis involving the hip, ankle, or foot may be the first symptom. Some children may have mild constitutional symptoms such as malaise, loss of appetite, or mild fever in early stage of the disease. These symptoms may be relatively more common in developing countries.

Sites along the back, pelvic bones, sacroiliac joints, and the chest may be tender due to the presence of **enthesitis** (see Chapter 15). Some children feel pain or tenderness at the bony prominence in front of the knee, located an inch or so below the knee cap (the tibial tubercle), or heel swelling and tenderness (due to Achilles tendonitis and plantar fasciitis) (see Figure 6).

Spondyloarthropathies

AS belongs to a family of diseases that may affect the spine and other joints, and also share many overlapping clinical features. This group of diseases are called spondyloarthropathies, and they are discussed in more detail in Chapter 17.

5
Exercise and physical therapy

Regular exercises are of fundamental importance in the successful long-term management of AS. They help maintain or improve posture, chest expansion, and spinal mobility, they improve health status, and they prevent or minimize deformity. Recreational exercise improves pain and stiffness, and exercising your back eases pain and improves function. Doing some recreational exercise at least 30 minutes per day and back exercises at least 5 days per week will improve your health status. Sports and recreational activities are discussed in more detail in Chapter 12.

Formal physiotherapy is helpful, especially as a source of information about proper posture, appropriate exercises and recreational sports, and the need for maintaining a regular exercise program. At least a couple of sessions at a physical therapy unit to learn these things from a physical therapist are recommended. A yearly follow-up by a physiotherapist can check that you are still performing these exercises appropriately, and also keep records of any improvement or worsening in physical posture, and range of motion of your joints and spine.

An exercise program of stretching and strengthening is needed to keep the muscles strong and the spine mobile and erect, and to retain good range of movement of certain joints, particularly hip and shoulder joints. Gentle stretching exercises ease stiffness and help prevent postural changes, and muscle-strengthening exercises help in retaining proper posture. Passive stretching of the hip joints increases their range of movement and thus improves function and posture.

Most people with AS feel too stiff to exercise in the morning, although taking a warm bath before exercising tends to ease this discomfort. Choose a time of the day that works best for you.

The use of large Swiss therapeutic exercise balls and group exercise sessions that include hydrotherapy are enjoyable and very helpful. In some European countries, professionally supervised special physiotherapy and hydrotherapy group sessions for AS patients have been organized by AS patient organizations. Randomized controlled trials have shown that physiotherapy with disease education is effective in the treatment of people with AS, and group physical therapy is cost-effective compared to individualized therapy.

Therapeutic exercises must be tailored to your degree of spinal mobility or involvement, you should do them routinely once or twice daily. Even though you may not be able to do them all daily, you should do at least some of them each day. Most people who comply with a comprehensive management program that depends upon a lifetime of daily exercises can maintain satisfactory spinal mobility, and can continue to lead full and productive lives.

Even with optimal treatment, some people will develop a stiff spine, but they will remain functional if the spine fuses in an upright position.

Swimming

Swimming is an ideal exercise for those who enjoy it, because it gently uses all the muscles and is very relaxing. It provides aerobic exercise to enhance general fitness and enhance lung capacity. A warm or even hot pool is generally most comfortable. A heated swimming pool or spa helps to decrease pain and stiffness, and therefore allows you to perform exercises when it might otherwise be impossible because of the pain. Low-impact exercises in the water (swimming and water aerobics) and stationary bicycling can help improve exercise capability, muscle strength, and range of motion.

Regular free-style swimming is considered to be one of the best exercises for people with AS, but if your neck is rigid it may be difficult to swim free-style. Using a snorkel may be helpful, provided you swim only under observation and near the edge of a swimming pool if it is deep. This precaution is necessary because someone with limited breathing capacity may not be able to blow the water out effectively if it inadvertently enters the snorkel tube.

You should be very careful not to slip on wet surfaces in the pool area, and it is also wise to avoid diving.

Application of heat

A warm shower or application of local heat may promote relaxation and help in passive stretching of tight muscles. You should not apply local heat to an area for more than 15 minutes at a time. Avoid areas overlying artificial joints. Keep the temperature setting of the heating pad at low or medium level, never on high setting. Do not lie on a heating pad to apply heat to your back, otherwise you will increase the risk of burn due to decreased blood circulation in the area that results from pressure of your body weight.

Spinal extension and deep breathing exercises

You can perform spinal extension exercises by lying face down on your front and then stretching your arms out at shoulder level and raising your chest, shoulders, arms, and head off the bed as far as possible (Figure 6). Hold your body in that position for about 5 seconds and then relax, and repeat the exercise about 20 times.

The chest expansion exercise is performed by lying on your back, clasping your hands behind your

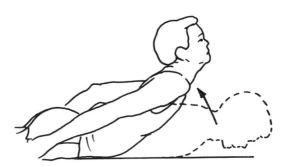

Figure 6

head, and extending your elbows outwards towards the bed while taking a deep breath. Hold the breath for a count of 10 before exhaling and relaxing for about 10 seconds. Repeat the exercise about 20 times. Give up smoking, in order to prevent its adverse effects on the lungs and heart.

You can combine the spinal extension and chest expansion by performing corner push-ups, in which you face a corner and place your hands on the opposing walls at shoulder height. Then bend your elbows to lean forward towards the corner with your head, neck, and spine fully extended, knees fully stretched and heels touching the ground (Figure 7). Take in a deep breath during this maneuver. After a count of 10, exhale while returning to the upright position. Repeat the exercise about 20 times, up to 3 times daily if possible.

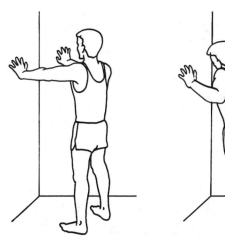

Figure 7

Muscle-strengthening and stretching exercises

Exercises to strengthen the extensor muscles of the back and hip can be performed in water or on land. You should try to achieve a functional range of motion of the hip and shoulder joint. Severe loss of motion of hip joints can be more disabling than the fused spine. Specific exercises such as daily stretching of involved joints may be needed to improve mobility of the back, hips, shoulders, or other involved joints (Figures 6–13). Physical exercises are needed to keep your joints from getting stiff, to regain muscle strength, and prevent muscle wasting and weakness.

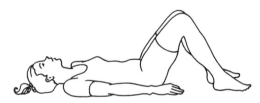

Figure 8a

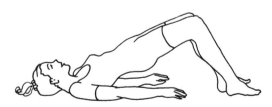

Figure 8b

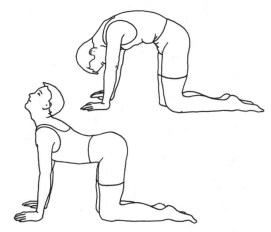

Figure 9a

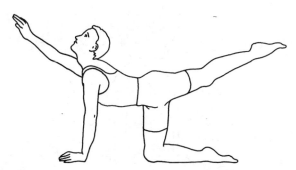

Figure 9b

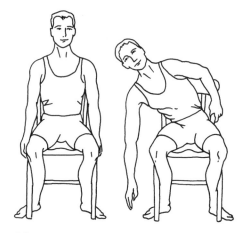

Figure 10a

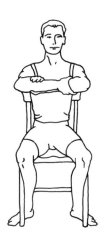

Figure 10b

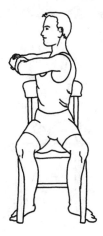

Figure 10c

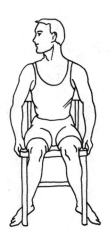

Figure 10d

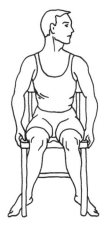

Figure 10e

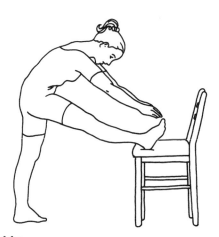

Figure 11a

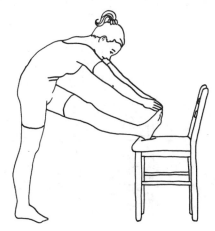

Figure 11b

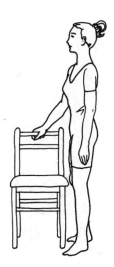

Figure 12a

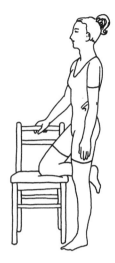

Figure 12b

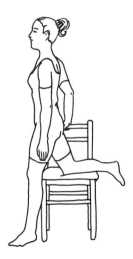

Figure 12c

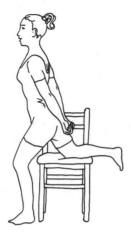

Figure 12d

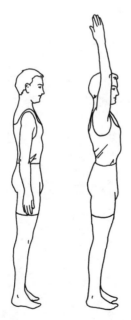

Figure 13a

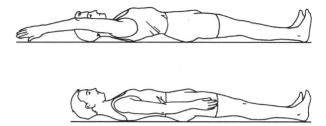

Figure 13b

6
Drug therapy

AS is a chronic disease, and there is currently no preventive measure or cure for it. There is no special diet, and there is no convincing scientific evidence that any specific food has anything to do with triggering the onset of AS or increasing its severity. A balanced diet rich in fresh fruits, and with adequate nutrients, such as calcium and vitamins, and a healthy lifestyle, without tobacco, alcohol or chemical addictions, are very important.

The severity of disease symptoms and the degree of joint involvement vary greatly from one person to another. Early accurate diagnosis and appropriate therapy may minimize years of pain and disability because with successful management it is often possible to minimize spinal deformity and slow down the progressive loss of mobility of spine and other affected joints. However, not everyone receives early diagnosis and appropriate medical management, and some people do not continue the recommended appropriate treatment. In such cases, posture and mobility are more likely to be permanently impaired.

The objectives of treatment—reducing pain and stiffness, maintaining erect posture, and preserving mobility—can only be achieved if the patient takes an active part. Continuing care and proper medical supervision and follow-up are critical. People with AS need a kind, caring and considerate doctor with a good bedside manner, who gives patients ample time, provides care and emotional support, and empathizes with their suffering. Because AS is a chronic (long-lasting) illness, it is to your advantage to have good relationships with your healthcare providers.

How effective is drug treatment?

Several drugs are used in treating AS. They do not cure the disease, but most minimize pain and help maintain mobility and function. The information provided below is only a guideline. You should ask your doctor and pharmacist about how and when to take any prescribed drugs and about their potential untoward effects.

NSAIDs

Non-steroidal anti-inflammatory drugs (NSAIDs), other than aspirin, are most often used in doses sufficient to reduce pain and suppress inflammation. The medicine must be taken as prescribed: you must take the full anti-inflammatory dose of NSAIDs during the active phase of the disease. Your health-care provider should emphasize this, because otherwise people may not realize how important it is and use the drugs only occasionally, for their pain-relieving (analgesic) effect.

Table 1 Some well-known NSAIDs*

Generic name	Brand name
Celecoxib	Celebrex
Choline magnesium trisalicylate	Trilisate
Diclofenac	Voltaren, Cataflam
Diclofenac sodium plus misoprostol	Arthrotec
Diflunisal	Dolobid
Disalcid	Salsalate
Etodolac	Lodine
Flurbiprofen	Ansaid
Ibuprofen	Motrin
Indomethacin	Indocid, Indocin
Ketoprofen	Orudis, Oruvail
Ketorolac tromethamnine	Toradol
Meloxicam	Mobic
Nabumetone	Relafen
Naproxen	Naprosyn, Naprelan
Naproxen sodium	Anaprox
Oxaprozin	Daypro
Piroxicam	Feldene
Rofecoxib	Vioxx
Sulindac	Clinoril
Tolmetin	Tolectin
Valdecoxib	Bextra

* The brand names given here are the ones used in the US and may vary
in different parts of the world. Other NSAIDs that are used relatively
infrequently in the US include fenoprofen (Nalfon), mefenamic acid
(Ponstel), and meclofenamate (Meclomen). The NSAIDs not available in
the US include nimesulide, tenoxicam, tiaprofenic acid, and
phenylbutazone.

More than 25 different NSAIDs are now available (Table 1). They are not all equally effective,
and not all of them may be officially approved by
drug-regulating agencies for use in AS in various
countries. Responses to them differ, as do their
untoward effects. The drug that best controls the
inflammation and pain may not be the first one that

your doctor tries; a trial period may be needed to find the most effective NSAID for you.

It is important to emphasize that in most instances the NSAID does not totally relieve pain and stiffness; an 80% pain relief, for example, may be a good enough result. You may need to take the NSAID for a few days before you can tell whether or not it is helping. Phenylbutazone (Butazolidin), one of the first NSAIDs, offers good relief of symptoms, but it is not generally used now because there is a potential risk of bone marrow toxicity.

Some NSAIDs need to be taken several times a day, but many longer-acting ones can be taken once or twice daily, which makes it easier for people to take the correct dose. In the last few years, three NSAIDs—ibuprofen (Motrin, Advil, Rufen, Excedrin, Nuprin), naproxen (Aleve, Anaprox), and ketoprofen (Actron, Orudis)—have become available over the counter in the US, so one can buy them without a doctor's prescription. Although these NSAIDs may relieve minor aches and pains, people with AS and related diseases need to take higher doses under a doctor's supervision.

With appreciable relief of back pain and stiffness at night, you should be able to get more restful sleep. Some people may benefit from the addition of a low dose (up to 30 mg nightly) of amitriptyline (Elavil), but it may cause some untoward effects, such as dry mouth and daytime drowsiness.

NSAIDs are relatively safe drugs, but the most common side-effects are stomach irritation, heartburn (caused by stomach acid flowing back into the esophagus), indigestion, and ulcers in the stomach or duodenum. There is an increased risk of gastrointestinal bleeding from ulcers, especially among people over the age of 60. Other risk factors include previous peptic ulcer disease. You should only take one NSAID at a time, in an adequate dose; using more than one NSAID at the same time increases the risk of side-effects without providing any additive benefit.

Many of the NSAIDs need to be taken with meals, not on an empty stomach, to avoid heartburn. Additional measures needed to control heartburn include:

- avoid foods and beverages, including alcohol that affect the sphincter between the esophagus and the stomach, or irritate the esophagus lining
- avoid lying down within 2 hours after eating
- raise the head of your bed about 6 inches (15 cm)
- stop smoking, if you are a smoker
- lose weight, if you are overweight.

If you have any acute abdominal pain, severe cramps or burning, vomiting, diarrhea, or black tarry stools, seek medical attention promptly.

Medicines called **H2-blockers** are more effective than antacids to treat acid indigestion, heartburn, and ulcer pain. These drugs include cimetidine (Tagamet), ranitidine (Zantac), famotidine (Pepcid), and nizatidine (Axid). Another group of drugs called **proton pump inhibitors** are even more effective; these drugs include esomeprazole (Nexium), omeprazole (Prilosec), and lansoprazole (Prevacid)

Some of the NSAIDs may impair the function of blood cells called platelets, thereby increasing your susceptibility to bruising or bleeding from cuts. They can also sometimes cause fluid retention and mild increase in blood pressure, or some blunting of the effect of drugs used to treat high blood pressure. On rare occasions there may be adverse effects on kidney or liver function, and a decrease in white or red blood cell count or other signs of bone marrow suppression. Some NSAIDs, indomethacin in particular, can cause headache, drowsiness, and some impairment of cognitive functions (a 'spaced-out' feeling), especially in elderly people. NSAIDs should not usually be taken during pregnancy or while breast-feeding.

COX-2 specific NSAIDs

Cyclo-oxygenase (COX) is a naturally occurring enzyme that exists in two forms, COX1 and COX2. COX1 can be considered the good enzyme because it helps in keeping intact the lining of the stomach and duodenum, in maintaining normal flow of blood through the kidneys, and in normal platelet stickiness and aggregation. If not enough COX1 is produced, the intestinal lining becomes vulnerable to ulceration and bleeding may occur. There may also be impairment of kidney and platelet function. COX2, the other variant of the enzyme, plays a role in pain and inflammation, and its production is stimulated by inflammatory disease, infection, or injury.

The traditional non-selective NSAIDs work by blocking the production of COX1 as well as COX2, which is why their side-effects include heartburn and stomach ulcers. However, three COX2-specific (or selective) NSAIDs are now available: **celecoxib** (Celebrex), **valdecoxib** (Bextra), and **rofecoxib** (Vioxx).

They offer a new strategy for the management of pain and inflammation since they are much safer on the stomach and duodenum, as far as ulcer risk is concerned, and can be taken with or without food. Moreover, they do not impair platelet function. Celecoxib has been studied in people with AS and is found to be as effective as ketoprofen, the compared NSAID.

However, the COX2-specific NSAIDs are no more effective than the conventional NSAIDs, and like them, may cause fluid retention, some increase in blood pressure, or potential impairment of kidney function. Women who are pregnant or are breastfeeding should not take them.

Sulfasalazine

Sulfasalazine (Azulfidine, Salazopyrin) may be effective in AS patients who have peripheral arthritis unresponsive to NSAIDs. It is one of the so-called disease-modifying anti-rheumatic drugs (DMARDs), also referred to simply as disease-modifying drugs or **slow-acting anti-rheumatic drugs**. These drugs may slow down or perhaps stop the progress of inflammatory arthritis in some people, but it may take a few months (which is why they are called slow-acting drugs).

Sulfasalazine is taken with food or a glass of milk, and is available as enteric-coated tablets to decrease the chance of stomach upset. The dose should start with one tablet daily in the evening for the first week, twice daily for the second week, three tablets daily (one in the morning and two in the evening) for the third week, and then two tablets twice daily. Only after taking the full dose of 4–6 tablets per day for 4–6 months will you know whether it is going to be of any help.

Sulfasalazine may be useful in controlling peripheral arthritis of AS, but has no appreciable influence on purely axial (spinal) disease or on peripheral enthesitis. Because it is frequently effective against inflammatory bowel disease and psoriasis, it may be especially useful for AS associated with those diseases. However, approximately 20% of patients stop the treatment because of side-effects, which include nausea, stomach upset, abdominal bloating, headaches, skin rashes, and mouth ulcers. On rare occasions sulfasalazine may cause liver problems and abnormal white blood-cell counts due to bone marrow suppression, and that's why your blood count and liver function must be regularly monitored if you are taking this drug.

Methotrexate

People with AS with severe peripheral joint involvement which does not respond to NSAIDs or sulfasalazine have sometimes responded to weekly oral **methotrexate** (Rheumatrex) therapy. Methotrexate and other immunosuppressants are used in the treatment of chronic inflammatory arthritis, such as rheumatoid arthritis and psoriatic arthritis resistant to conventional therapy. It is also a relatively slow-acting anti-rheumatic drug, and anyone taking it should not expect a quick response. Like sulfasalazine, methotrexate is not a pain reliever, but it will help to relieve pain if it can first heal or control the underlying inflammation that contributes to the pain.

It is usually well tolerated but can cause loss of appetite, nausea, diarrhea, hair loss, cough, and bruising. You should tell your doctor right away if you get a dry cough, fever, or difficulty in breathing. Liver and blood tests and a chest X-ray are advised before starting the drug, and the treatment is monitored for side-effects by liver tests and blood counts. Methotrexate is not suitable for people with liver and lung disease, alcoholism, an abnormal blood count, or active infection.

Methotrexate may temporarily reduce fertility in men and women, but the risk appears to be very low, as far as we can tell at present. In men there is a theoretical risk of sperm damage. Therefore, it is sensible to wait for 6 months after discontinuing the drug before attempting to start a baby. This allows for drug washout and avoids any theoretical risk of fetal exposure.

Methotrexate may cause birth defects if taken during pregnancy. The most vulnerable period is between 6 and 8 weeks of pregnancy at a critical methotrexate dose of more than 10 mg weekly. Breastfeeding should also be avoided while a woman is taking methotrexate.

Corticosteroids

Oral corticosteroids are powerful anti-inflammatory drugs but cause a number of side-effects, including osteoporosis (discussed in Chapter 9), weight gain, thinning of the skin, cataract in the eye, elevation of blood pressure, raised blood sugar, poor wound healing, and increased susceptibility to infections. They have no therapeutic value in the long-term management of the musculoskeletal aspects of AS because of their serious side-effects, and they do not stop the progression of the disease. Local corticosteroid injection, however, is quite helpful in controlling persistent joint inflammation and enthesitis. The benefit of injection into the sacroiliac joints is currently being evaluated.

New drug treatments

TNF-based therapy

Results of clinical trials now provide encouraging evidence of a prompt and dramatic improvement in symptoms for patients with a variety of ailments when treated with drugs that block the action of a natural substance in the body called **tumor necrosis factor alpha** (**TNF**, for short). The diseases that can be treated include severe forms of rheumatoid arthritis, juvenile idiopathic arthritis (also called juvenile rheumatoid arthritis), and many other inflammatory diseases, including Crohn's disease, that are resistant to conventional therapy.

Anti-TNF therapy has now been found to be very effective in severe AS, psoriatic arthritis, and other spondyloarthropathies that are unresponsive to conventional therapy. However, it can have serious side-effects, and whether it is safe as a long-term therapy also remains to be seen.

What is TNF?

TNF is a **cytokine** produced by certain inflammatory cells. Cytokines are messenger proteins that play a key role in the body's immune response by controlling the production of other substances involved in inflammation. The effect of TNF is to promote inflammation and also to help cells to heal or repair themselves. It attaches to a cell surface protein called TNF receptor on the cells belonging to the immune system. This receptor draws TNF into the cell to exert its effect. When cells have enough TNF, they release some of their TNF receptors into the bloodstream. These released TNF receptors mop up any excess TNF that is circulating in the bloodstream or is present in the tissues.

The original reason for calling this substance 'tumor necrosis factor' was that is could induce destruction (necrosis) of cancerous tumors in laboratory studies. When it was first discovered it was tested for its ability to induce destruction of cancerous tumors in animals and later in cancer patients. However, doses large enough to shrink tumors caused serious toxic reactions in cancer patients.

What is anti-TNF therapy?

If too much TNF is produced, it can damage healthy tissues and contribute to a variety of ailments such as toxic shock. One way the scientists could prevent this in laboratory animals was by administering decoy TNF receptors that can capture excess TNF, or by treatment with anti-TNF antibodies. However, when such anti-TNF therapies were tested in human patients with toxic shock, the results were disappointing.

TNF is also involved in triggering the inflammatory response in many chronic inflammatory diseases such as rheumatoid arthritis and AS. Laboratory animals genetically altered to produce too much of this substance develop arthritis, and administering anti-TNF antibody to these animals can prevent the development of this arthritis.

In 1992, 20 people with rheumatoid arthritis were treated with the anti-TNF antibody called infliximab (Remicade), a genetically engineered hybrid molecule made by combining human and mouse proteins. This study provided clear-cut evidence of the effectiveness and relative safety of infliximab. Additional trials have now established infliximab as a new treatment for severe rheumatoid arthritis and Crohn's disease, although the therapy does not provide a cure. Infliximab is now known to be very effective in treating severe AS and related spondyloarthropathies which do not respond to conventional therapy. The drug is given by intravenous infusion every month (or possibly every other month), after the first two infusions which are given 2 weeks apart.

Another genetically engineered, human-derived molecule called etanercept (Enbrel) has a similar anti-TNF effect. It is composed of components of the normal human TNF receptor attached to a normal human blood protein called IgG1. It acts as a decoy TNF receptor that snags and neutralizes excess TNF and keeps it from binding the TNF receptors on cell surfaces. Etanercept is supplied as a sterile white, preservative-free powder, which must be stored in the refrigerator. For use, it is dissolved in sterile water and injected under the skin twice weekly.

The possible down side

Infliximab and etanercept are called biologic response modifiers, or biologicals for short. They work quite rapidly, and are very effective in treating many types of arthritis resistant to conventional therapy. The systemic features of aching and fatigue tend to resolve very quickly, making people feel a lot better. However, 20% of people with rheumatoid arthritis, the disease in which biologicals have been studied most, do not respond, suggesting that other promoters of inflammation may be at work in such patients.

Anti-TNF therapy is very costly (up to $13 000 a year). Another major concern is that because these drugs are so new, long-term scrutiny for their possible side-effects is needed. TNF plays a key role in the body's defense against infection by promoting inflammation and helping cells repair themselves. Long-term anti-TNF drug therapy might leave people vulnerable to potentially serious infections. In addition, as with other therapies aimed at modifying the body's immune response, there is a theoretical possibility that anti-TNF therapy may promote malignant disease (cancer) in the long run. Doctors and patients must carefully weigh the present advantages against future, as yet unknown, side-effects.

Other potential new therapies

Experimental drug therapies under study for possible benefit in the treatment of refractory AS include **thalidomide** and **pamidronate**; the latter needs to be given into the vein as an infusion.

Most doctors now believe that radiation treatment of the spine has no place in the modern management of AS, because of potentially serious and even fatal side-effects, including cancer and bone marrow failure, which may occur many years after the course of radiation therapy. However, in German-speaking countries, radium treatment that gives only mild radiation is still occasionally used at a few centers for treating severe AS if NSAIDs do not help. The treatment may take the form of radon gas inhalation, or a bath (radon dissolved in water) at some spa centers, or injection of radioactive high-purity radium chloride.

The present author has no experience in this area and would not recommend this form of treatment, in part because of concerns about its long-term safety, and because alternative, effective and relatively safer methods of treatment are available for managing patients unresponsive to NSAIDs.

Storage of medications

Keep all medications out of reach of children, even if the bottles have 'child-resistant caps', because these caps are not 'child proof'. Do not store drugs in the bathroom cabinet because humidity and heat may impair their effectiveness. Discard medicines when they reach their expiry date shown on the bottle. Make sure that the expiry date is shown on the bottle when you buy any medicines.

7

Nontraditional (complementary, or alternative) therapy

Complementary and alternative healthcare remedies have lately become more popular. The American population spends more than $1 billion a year on nontraditional treatments or folk remedies for arthritis. People use such treatments for many reasons, such as lack of adequate relief with many conventional arthritis medicines, or their untoward effects. Another reason is that many conventional medical and surgical treatments are quite costly. Moreover, arthritis treatment attracts charlatans peddling 'miracle cures'.

Unlike conventional medicines, nutritional supplements and herbal preparations are not regulated by agencies such as the US Food and Drug Administration (FDA). People are therefore using many of these substances without any certainty about their precise strength, composition, and dose, and without scientifically valid proof of their safety or effectiveness. Moreover, some practitioners providing complementary medicine do not need to have a license or other proof of their competency to prescribe such remedies or procedures. Some forms of complementary medicine may also be expensive, and it is not usually covered by health insurance.

The use of many of the complementary and alternative treatments is based on mostly anecdotal evidence, mostly from individuals who report their own successful use of the treatment. Scientific methods should be applied to establish the validity of the anecdotal evidence.

Sometimes people benefit from nontraditional remedies because of the **placebo effect**, and on other occasions they may experience coincidental 'cure' because many rheumatic diseases can have cyclical spontaneous disease flare-ups and remissions. It is tempting to credit relief of symptoms to the complementary medicine that, just by chance, was started when the disease was beginning to go into remission, even though the medicine may really have had no effect on the disease.

A Canadian survey of people with osteoarthritis found that many of them had used a variety of complementary therapies, but only 30% of them had discussed this with their doctors. These therapies included chiropractic treatment, acupuncture, massage therapy, yoga, homeopathy, naturopathic remedies, and nutritional supplements and multivitamins. Three-quarters had used vitamins.

Anyone with limited spinal mobility due to AS should avoid manipulation of their back or neck by **chiropractors** and masseurs, because it can be dangerous. Such treatment have sometimes inadvertently led to spinal fractures and neurological complications.

Diets

Elimination diets require you to stop eating certain foods. One investigator has suggested the possible beneficial effect of a **low-starch diet** involving a reduced intake of bread, potatoes, cakes, and pasta in the management of AS. However, this diet has not been scientifically evaluated and there has been no independent scientifically valid confirmation of its overall benefit, so it is therefore not recommended.

Nutritional supplements that contain vitamins C, E and A, and omega-3 fatty acids are being studied as possible treatments for arthritis. Glucosamine and chondroitin sulfate supplements are also under study to establish if they have any beneficial effect in osteoarthritis of the knee. S-Adenosylmethionine (SAM-e, pronounced Sam-ee), a compound that occurs naturally in all human tissues, is another supplement that is being studied as a possible therapy for osteoarthritis. It has been used in Europe for years as a prescription medication for arthritis and depression, and it became available in the US as an over-the-counter supplement in March 1999.

Homeopathy

Homeopathy uses extremely diluted preparations of natural substances, such as plants and minerals, and scientists are skeptical about its effectiveness. A recent study of the homeopathic treatment with 'Formica ruta' concluded that it is not effective in AS.

Traditional Chinese medicine

The ancient **taditional Chinese system of medicine (TCM)** includes herbal and nutritional supplements, meditation, acupuncture, and restorative physical exercises and massage.

Herbs are the basis for many traditional medicines, such as aspirin, morphine, and digitalis; and practitioners of some complementary therapies believe that certain herbs have anti-inflammatory effects. Many of the herbal therapies that are now used in complementary or alternative medicine were used by the mainstream medical profession up until the early part of the twentieth century in the western world. Many of them are still considered mainstream medicine in some poorer regions of the world that lack modern healthcare and its effective therapies. Some herbs contain powerful and potentially toxic substances that can interfere with other medications that you may be taking, so you should talk to your doctor before taking any herbal preparation.

The regular practice of **meditation** helps you to enter a deeply restful and relaxed state, with a reduction in the body's stress response, slowing of brain waves and heartbeat, and decrease in muscle tension.

A doctor with AS has reported his personal experience with **Tai Chi** (Koh, 1982), a traditional Chinese mind–body relaxation exercise system.

Acupuncture is based on the Chinese concept of balanced Qi (pronounced *chee*), or vital energy, that flows throughout the body via 12 main and 8 secondary pathways (called meridians), accessed through the more than 2000 acupuncture points on the human body. It is one of the oldest medical procedures in the world, originating in China more than 2000 years ago. It is believed to remove the imbalances of Yin (negative energy and forces in the universe and human body) and Yang (positive energy). This brings the body into balance, keeps the normal flow of the vital energy Qi unblocked, and restores health to the mind and body.

Acupuncture became widely known in the US in 1971 when *New York Times* reporter James Reston wrote about how doctors in China eased his abdominal pain after surgery by puncturing the skin with hair-thin needles at particular locations. Although the mechanism of action is unclear, stimulation of acupuncture points may lead to release by the brain and spinal cord (via the endorphin system) of opium-like molecules (neurotransmitters and neurohormones), that help to modulate pain; the same can happen also after vigorous exercise.

Acupuncture could work due to its placebo effect. It has been shown that a real drug, naloxone (which inhibits endorphin-producing cells in the brain), can reverse pain relief obtained by placebo (sham) painkiller; this indicates that in some cases placebo works via the endorphin system. The Chinese claim that acupuncture also leads to biochemical changes that may stimulate healing and promote general well-being.

The World Health Organization (WHO), which is the health branch of the United Nations, lists more than 40 conditions for which acupuncture is used, including nonspecific back and neck pain, and arthritis. This is based on mostly anecdotal evidence, mostly from people who report their own successful use of the treatment. Scientific studies are under way to establish the validity of this anecdotal evidence of the potential benefit of acupuncture in some forms of arthritis (see NIH, 1998).

Other therapies

Hypnosis can also be used to promote relaxation and help you cope better with pain. Another way of achieving a restful and relaxed state is by **guided imagery**, which involves creating a vivid and pleasant mental picture. For example, you might see yourself sitting on a beach on a warm day, looking at the waves and hearing them pounding on the shore. A related method called **bio-feedback** involves using various machines that monitor one's body temperature, heart rate, breathing patterns, and other bodily functions, and provide feedback that helps you to learn how to produce these effects and a feeling of relaxation voluntarily, without the need for machine monitors.

Holistic medicine deals with an integrated comprehensive overview of a physical, mental, emotional, and spiritual being; practitioners may suggest therapies based on the whole person, including spiritual and mental aspects, not just the specific part of the body being treated. They may advise changes in diet, lifestyle, and physical activity to help treat your condition.

Transcutaneous electrical nerve stimulation (**TENS**) requires passing an electric current to nerve cells through electrodes placed on the skin. This technique is of no value for people with AS.

Bee and snake venom are used by some alternative practitioners who claim that bee venom relieves the symptoms of rheumatoid arthritis because it contains certain enzymes, and stimulates the body to produce more corticosteroids. This treatment is potentially dangerous for about 10% of the population who have mild, severe, or even fatal allergic reactions to insect venom. Snake venom is toxic and there is little scientific support for its use in treating arthritis.

Ayurveda, the traditional Indian system of medicine, is also not effective in AS.

The wearing of **copper bracelets**, according to folk lore, allows trace amounts of copper to be absorbed through the skin and neutralize toxic molecules called free radicals that can otherwise damage tissues. These bracelets appear to be harmless, but there is no scientific basis for their medical benefit.

The use of **magnets** as a possible therapy for joint aches and pains, and their possible untoward effects, is being investigated.

Aromatherapy practitioners believe that oils derived from plant extracts and resins can help treat various illnesses when inhaled or massaged into the skin.

Dimethyl sulfoxide (DMSO) is an industrial solvent similar to turpentine, and the industrial-grade DMSO sold in hardware stores may contain harmful contaminants. Some people believe that DMSO or its breakdown product **methyl sulfonyl methane** (MSM) can relieve pain and reduce swelling when rubbed on the skin, but rheumatologists do not recommend its use.

In the end it is important to emphasize again that there is no rigorous scientific evidence to support the use of these complementary and alternative therapies by people with AS.

Finding out about complementary therapies

There are many quacks preying on the pain and suffering of vulnerable or desperate people. These quacks may promote or promise questionable and sometimes outright dangerous treatments as 'cures', and may even harm people not only financially but also medically, by keeping them away from effective therapies.

The National Center for Complementary and Alternative Medicine (NCCAM) recommends that people should take the following steps before trying any complementary therapy:

- Talk to your doctor first. Some forms of complementary therapy that you plan to take may interfere with your current treatments or affect other illnesses that you may have. Moreover, always let your doctor know if you are already taking any complementary therapy because some therapies may potentially interact with the medicines that you may be currently taking as prescribed by your doctor.
- Ask the healthcare provider or the complementary therapy practitioner about the expected beneficial results, risks, costs and length of treatment.
- Check the credentials of the practitioner. Research the expertise of the practitioner or

salesperson associated with a given treatment.
Check with your local or state business bureau
if you are going to buy a product from a
business.

- Testimonials of other people with arthritis who
have tried a complementary or alternative treatment cannot prove how safe or effective the
treatment will be for others.

- Obtain objective scientific information about it
at a library or through reliable Internet sources
(see below).

Using the Internet

Doctors should encourage their patients to be well
informed about their disease; patients will comply
better with treatment overall if they are properly
informed and understand the rationale for their
treatment (Brus *et al.*, 1997). The Internet-savvy
patient's ability to obtain information need not
adversely impact the patient/physician relationship.
Much useful information can be obtained from the
Internet. However, you should be selective and not
believe everything that 'washes ashore while you are
surfing the Net' (Suarez-Almazor *et al.*, 2001).
There is a lot of misinformation out there too, and
this can be harmful.

You can find objective scientific information from
reliable sources, such as the National Institutes of
Health (NIH) and MEDLINE Plus at *www.nlm.nih.
gov/medlineplus*. Appendix 1 gives contact details for
some AS organizations, which are also a useful
source of information (see also page 152).

8
Surgical treatment

Joint replacement (arthroplasty)

Total hip arthroplasty (THA) gives very good results, and to a large extent prevents partial or total disability from severe hip disease. People who are about to undergo THA should be in good general and dental health.

Infection can be a serious complication, but with advances in the use of antibiotics and other technical aspects, the occurrence of infections has been markedly reduced in recent years. Bacteria can travel through the blood and infect a total joint implant, both in the early postoperative period and for some years following implantation; the most critical period is the first 2 years after joint replacement. Dental and endoscopic procedures can cause temporary circulation of bacteria in the blood, so people with artificial joints undergoing these procedures (e.g. cystoscopy and colonoscopy) may need prophylactic antibiotics to minimize the risk of infection affecting the replaced joint.

Prophylaxis

People who are not allergic to penicillin should be given amoxicillin 2 grams by mouth 1 hour before a dental procedure (or cefazolin 1 gram or ampicillin 2 grams by injection 1 hour before the procedure if the patient cannot take oral medications). People who are allergic to penicillin can be given clinda-mycin 600 mg by mouth 1 hour before the dental procedure, or by injection if they cannot take oral medications. No second doses are recommended.

The American Heart Association's suggested regimen is 3 grams of amoxicillin 1 hour before and 1.5 grams 6 hours after the initial dose. For someone allergic to penicillin, then erythromycin may be given, 1 gram 1 hour before dental treatment and 500 milligrams 6 hours after the first dose. Clindamycin may be used an alternative.

Other surgical procedures

Severe spinal forward curvature (kyphosis) used to occur in some people with severe AS, but its occurrence should now be very uncommon if the disease is diagnosed at an early stage and treated appropriately. Severe kyphosis can be surgically corrected for someone so bent that they cannot look straight ahead, or are hardly able to eat. However, this surgery carries a relatively high risk of paraplegia. If surgery is too risky, special prism spectacles can help people to look ahead while walking, but they are not easy to use. Spinal surgery may also be needed for stabilization of spinal fracture.

Heart complications, such as leaky heart valve or severe slowing of the heart may require valve replacement or the placement of a cardiac (heart) pacemaker. Scarring (fibrosis) and cavity (cyst) formation in the upper part (apex) of the lung are rare complications of AS that are not easy to manage; surgical removal of tissue may sometimes be required.

Anesthesia in people with AS

The anesthesiologist may have difficulty in passing a breathing tube down the trachea (windpipe) so that the airway can be maintained during general anes-thesia for surgery. This is a potential problem in anyone with a rigid spine, especially if you also have forward stooping of the neck and a reduced jaw-opening capacity. An instrument called a **fiber optic laryngoscope** helps in putting the breathing tube down the trachea. However, someone with extreme neck deformity may require a **tracheostomy**. Post-surgical lung complications are also more likely, owing to severely restricted chest wall movement.

Lumbar spinal anesthesia or other alternatives to general anesthesia, such as **epidural** anesthesia, may be possible for some surgical procedures (e.g. total hip joint replacement surgery). However, lumbar puncture for spinal anesthesia is often not possible in AS patients with a fused lumbar spine.

Do not assume that healthcare providers are fully aware of all the limitations due to AS. You should discuss any concerns or apprehensions with the surgeon, and arrange a preoperative consultation with the anesthesiologist. The anesthesiologist should examine you beforehand to find out your limitations, and also allay any concerns you may have. This should preferably be done in your hospital room, before you are taken to the operating room, and before you are given the anesthetic premedications that dim your alertness of mind.

9
Some later manifestations

Osteoporosis

Osteoporosis (porous bone) is a very common accompaniment of aging and therefore a common condition, among the general population, but it poses particular problems for people with AS, as we will see later in the chapter. It is a major problem for close to 30 million US citizens, 80% of them women, although it is a potentially preventable illness. One out of 2 women and 1 in 8 men over the age of 50 will have an osteoporosis-related fracture in their lifetime.

Osteoporosis is characterized by low bone mass that leads to an increased susceptibility to fractures of the spine, hip, wrist, ribs, and other bones. It is often called the 'silent disease' because there may be no symptoms until the bones become so weak that a fall or sudden strain causes a fracture of one or more bones of the limbs or the spine. Fractures of the spinal vertebrae can be in the form of compression (collapse) fractures, and these may lead to loss of height, back pain, and the stooped posture called dowager's hump. In a patient with osteoporosis, usually an elderly woman, the hump occurs in the upper back (thoracic kyphosis), and the spinal curvature may look superficially like AS.

An average woman acquires 98% of her total skeletal bone mass by about age 20 and can lose up to 20% of her bone mass in the first 5 years after menopause. The best defense against developing osteoporosis in later life is to build strong bones during childhood and early adulthood by taking a balanced diet rich in calcium and vitamin D, following a healthy lifestyle with no smoking, and performing regular weight-bearing exercise.

Significant risk of osteoporosis has been reported in people of all ethnic backgrounds, but it is more common among whites and Asians, and white women after age 65 are twice as likely as African-American women to get fractures. Specialized bone density tests can detect osteoporosis before a fracture occurs, and can also predict your chances of bone fracture in the future. Tests conducted at appropriate intervals can measure rate of bone loss and monitor treatment benefit.

Osteoporosis is responsible for more than 1.5 million fractures annually in the US, with an estimated national direct expenditure (hospitals and nursing homes) of $14 billion annually (and rising). People over 50 years of age have an average 1 in 4 chance of dying in the year following a hip fracture, and among those who survive there is 1 in 4 chance that they will require long-term care afterward. A woman's risk of hip fracture is equal to her combined risk of breast, uterine, and ovarian cancer.

Osteoporosis is often thought of a disease of old people, or women past the age of menopause.

However, it can strike at a younger age in people with predisposing (risk) factors, which include a diet low in calcium; chronic use of certain medications (e.g. corticosteroids); being female, thin, or having a small frame; a family history of osteoporosis; an inactive lifestyle; smoking; excessive intake of alcohol; propensity to falls; anorexia nervosa, and (for men) low testosterone levels.

Drug therapy for osteoporosis

Bisphosphonates such as **alendronate** (Fosamax) and **risedronate** (Actonel) are very helpful, and are more widely used than treatment with **calcitonin** (Miacalcin). Calcium tablets may be needed if the calcium intake in your diet needs to be supplemented.

For women after the menopause the female hormone **estrogen** helps to prevent or slow down osteoporosis. Brand names include Premarin (without progesterone), Prempro (with progesterone), Estratab (esterified estrogen), and others. **Raloxifene** (Evista) is the first in a new class of drugs called **selective estrogen receptor molecules** (SERMs) that slow bone loss like estrogens do, but without some of estrogen's untoward effects on the breast and uterus. Therefore, raloxifen can be an alernative choice for women at increased risk for cancer of the breast or uterus. However, like estrogens, it is associated with increased risk of blood clots and stroke.

Spinal fracture in AS

Recent studies indicate that osteoporosis can also occur in many people with AS in early stages of their disease. It can be a result of inflammation in the early stages of AS, as well as a result of immobility in the later stages of the disease. In advanced AS the spine usually has a low bone mass, i.e. it is **osteoporotic**. This structural deterioration, along with immobility due to bony fusion, makes the spine fragile and very susceptible to fracture.

People with AS are five times more likely to get spinal fractures than the general population. These fractures may follow a relatively minor trauma, especially in people with long-standing AS that has resulted in a fused spine. They usually affect the lower neck (cervical spine). The two commonest causes are falls and motor vehicle accidents.

The pain associated with spinal fractures may be overlooked, or wrongly attributed to exacerbation of the underlying AS. The best early clues to spinal fracture may be an acute or unexplained episode of back pain, even in the absence of a history of physical injury, that is aggravated by movement and may sometimes be associated with localized spinal tenderness.

There may be neurological signs and symptoms as a result of the fracture. The displaced ends of the fractured cervical spine (neck) compressing the spinal cord may cause **quadriplegia** (weakness or paralysis of all four limbs), the most dreaded complication of AS. Isolated or multiple vertebral compression fractures without displacement may also occur.

If you have a fused spine it is wise to carry a suitable **personalized information card**. The card should state that your spine, including your neck, is fused as a result of AS, and that you are therefore much more prone to spinal fracture due to any fall or motor vehicle accident, even after a relatively trivial injury. The card should include your name, address, and phone number, a photograph (including a picture showing the spinal deformity), your blood group type, a list of medicines you are taking, any allergy history, and contact details of your doctor.

Inflammation of the discs in the back (**spondylodiscitis**) may sometimes occur without any physical trauma or infection. This mostly occurs in the mid-thoracic spine, is usually without any symptoms, and is relatively more common in people with AS severe enough to involve the neck.

Neurological problems

As well as quadriplegia or paraplegia resulting from spinal fracture, other neurological problems may occur (although they are rare). For example, there may be a gradual loosening of a joint at the junction of the skull and the neck as a result of inflammation; this condition is called **spontaneous subluxation of the atlantoaxial joint**.

Rarely, patients with advanced AS may have problems resulting from gradual scarring of the covering at the lower end of the spine that entraps the lower spinal nerves. The resultant symptom complex is called **cauda equina syndrome.** (The name cauda equina means horsetail, so named because the lowermost spinal nerves slope downward as a bunch before they leave the vertebral column.) Symptoms may include urinary retention and incontinence, fecal incontinence due to decrease rectal tone, sexual dysfunction, saddle anesthesia (so called because of loss of skin sensation over the part we sit on), and pain and weakness of the legs.

Other problems

Some people may get kidney dysfunction due to treatment with NSAIDs or other drugs used to treat AS, especially if they have underlying kidney disease, perhaps due to diabetes or high blood pressure. A complication that has now become very rare, especially in North America, is amyloidosis of the kidneys, which used to be the most common cause of kidney dysfunction in patients with AS. Rare occurrence of IgA kidney disease (**glomeru-lonephritis**) has been reported in some countries.

The uncommon heart and lung complications have been mentioned previously (see pages 62–3).

10
A typical case history

Adam, a 26-year-old college student, was recently seen with back pain. He had been quite well up until 18 months ago, when he started having chronic low back pain and stiffness. He initially felt the pain in his buttocks for a few months, and then it progressed to involve the low back area as well, and was associated with back stiffness. Now his symptoms of back pain and stiffness are worsened by prolonged sitting, and at night, as well as when he wakes up in the morning. His back symptoms are worse when he first gets out of bed but they start easing up after about 40 minutes, or after physical activity or exercise, and after a hot shower. In the last 3 months Adam has noticed pain in the chest (rib cage) that is accentuated on coughing or sneezing.

He has no history of chronic diarrhea, skin disease, eye inflammation or injury to his back. His father was killed in a car accident at the age of 30, and he is an only child. His paternal uncle has had a stiff back and neck for many years.

On physical examination, Adam was found to have tenderness over sacroiliac joints, the lumbar spine, anterior chest wall, and right jaw joint (temporomadibular joint), as well as limitation of motion of his lumbar spine. His chest expansion on full inspiration was normal, and the rest of his physical examination was also normal.

Because these clinical findings indicated a strong probability of AS, an X-ray of the pelvis was ordered. The presence of bilateral sacroiliitis on the X-ray confirmed the diagnosis of AS.

He was prescribed an NSAID to be taken twice a day with food, and was encouraged to stay active, swim regularly if possible, and follow a regular exercise regimen. His illness was explained to him, and he was given counseling and provided with a pamphlet that gives further information about AS. Julian is computer-literate, so he was also given the Internet addresses of reputable self-help groups and organizations for AS patients.

When he was seen at a follow-up visit 2 weeks later, Adam's symptoms were already much better. Assessment of pain, physical function, spinal mobility (including chest expansion), duration of morning stiffness, presence of any inflamed peripheral joints, and enthesitis are critical elements that will be followed over time by the medical personnel caring for him. Laboratory tests, such as **C-reactive protein (CRP)** and **erythrocyte sedimentation rate (ESR)**, and occasionally musculoskeletal imaging (changes on X-ray pelvis and spine) will also help his doctors to assess and monitor the activity and severity of his disease.

Adam asked a lot of questions about AS and possible treatments, and he had already accessed many websites and other information sources.

Because he takes an intelligent interest in his disease, he is more likely to follow the recommended exercise program and to comply with his medication and follow-up schedule.

11
Living with ankylosing spondylitis: some hints

If you have physical limitations due to advanced AS, there are many devices to help perform daily tasks: walking canes, special chairs and desks, special shoes, and devices that assist in putting on socks or stockings and shoes, or for scratching or applying soap on the back, etc.

Avoiding falls

- Always wear a good pair of skid-resistant shoes.
- Use grab bars in the shower and toilets, shower seats, raised toilet seats, and floor lighting at night.
- Avoid slippery surfaces and loose carpets.

Posture

- It is important to sleep on a firm bed to maintain a good resting posture at night. You should preferably make a habit of sleeping on your back, to prevent the hip joints and the back from becoming bent (Figure 14a). Avoid a pillow

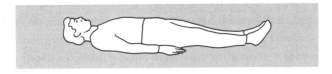

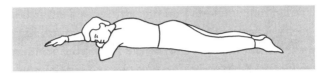

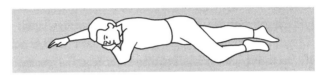

Figure 14 Recommended sleeping positions: (a) A flat sleeping position opposes the tendency of curvature. If your head would fall into over-extension because your thoracic spine is already curved, a small pillow of just the right thickness under the back of your head may make the position easier. Avoid too thick a pillow. (b) Lying 'face down' (on your stomach) is also a favorable position. (c) If lying on your front is no longer possible, a stable position lying on your side (the 'recovering position', is a good alternative.

under your knees because that will increase the tendency to muscle and tendon shortening.

- Avoid a saggy mattress or a waterbed. A suitable board (made of plywood or chipboard) can be put between the mattress and the bed frame to make the bed more firm.
- Avoid using a pillow if possible, or use one just thick enough to allow a horizontal position of the face to prevent pain from overextension of the neck.

- You should only lie on your side for short periods, if possible.
- You should also practice lying prone (with the face down), e.g. for 5 minutes or more before getting out of the bed in the morning, and also before going to bed at night (Figure 14b). Or you can lie on your back across your bed with your legs over the side and knees bent.
- People with AS need to practice good posture habits at all times, and should be taught about dynamic, resting, and occupational postures.

Dynamic posture

- Be aware of how you are standing, and try to maintain an erect tall posture, with the spine kept as straight as possible.
- Avoid any tendency to slump forward.
- Splints, braces and corsets are generally not helpful and are not advised. Some form of bracing may be necessary on rare occasions, e.g. after injury to the back or neck, but only on the recommendation of a doctor who is experienced in the management of AS patients.
- Perform appropriate muscle-strengthening exercises regularly, as advised by your doctor.

Occupational posture

- Analyze your habitual and work postures and modify your working positions to maintain a good posture. For example, a drafting table with tilting work surface (Figure 15) may be better than an ordinary office desk for writing and reading, and avoiding stress on the neck.

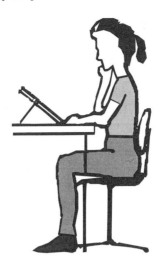

Figure 15

- Avoid physical activity that places prolonged strain on your back and neck muscles, and prolonged stooping or bending.
- Alternate between sitting and standing positions to perform jobs that take a long time to finish.
- Maintain a good posture while sitting, and avoid sitting for prolong periods, especially in low soft sofas and chairs.
- During your mid-day break at work, lie flat for a few minutes, and do some corner push-ups to stretch the back (Figure 7). Try to lie face down on your stomach for part of the time.
- A daily routine of deep breathing and spine motion/stretching exercises may minimize the fusion, and at least preserve better posture. Do

deep breathing exercises at frequent intervals during the day.

Thus proper sitting, sleeping, walking, and working positions, coupled with appropriate exercises, help maintain good posture and chest expansion. Because hip and shoulder joints are often affected, you should exercise the range of motion of these joints even before you observe any symptoms or limited motion there.

Family life

- People with AS generally have a very fulfilling and productive life. You can raise children just like anyone else because the disease usually does not interfere with family life.
- Fertility, pregnancy, and childbirth are usually normal.
- Although pregnancy does not usually affect the symptoms of AS, there may be restrictions on certain kinds of drug therapy during pregnancy and breast-feeding. You should discuss the use of any drug at these times with your doctor.
- Problems with family life may sometimes arise as a result of severe back pain, spinal deformity or limited spinal mobility; especially in women who have severe involvement of the hip joints with marked pain and limitation of joint movement. You should discuss these problems with your doctor. Patients with severe hip involvement benefit from total hip joint replacement surgery (see Chapter 8).
- A very useful and informative publication titled *Straight talk on spondylitis*, published by the

Spondylitis Association of America, is highly recommended for additional advice. It also discusses housework, dressing and grooming, child bearing and child care. See Appendix 1 for contact details.

Sports and recreational activities

- Sports and recreational activities that encourage good posture as well as arching of the back (extension) and rotation of the trunk are recommended. These include walking, hiking, swimming, tennis, badminton, cross-country skiing, and archery.
- Volleyball and basketball (with specially adapted rules) are excellent sports for people with AS as

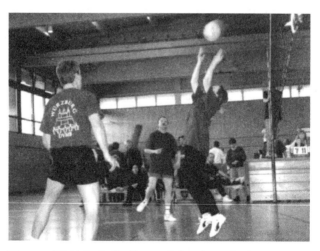

Figure 16 Volleyball with specially adapted rules as practised in local groups of AS organizations (here of the German AS society) is an excellent sport for people with AS as it combines movement with stretching.

they combine movement with stretching (Figure 16). However, not everyone can tolerate jarring activities.

- If you have neck involvement you need to be more careful, and follow safety instructions.
- Sports activities that require prolonged spinal flexion, including golfing, bowling, and long-distance cycling, may be inadvisable.
- Body contact sports (such as boxing, rugby, soccer, American football, and hockey), and downhill skiing, are also not recommended because of their greater potential for injury.
- Stationary bike exercises are good, but the handlebars must be properly adjusted so that you do not lean forward while exercising. This exercise is especially good for general cardiovascular conditioning, strengthening the leg muscles, and exercising the hip and knee joints.
- Aerobic exercises with machines that enhance back, leg, and shoulder extension are helpful, but you should avoid undue stress on the neck.

Car driving

- You may find difficulty driving if you have impaired mobility of your neck. In particular, it may be difficult to back the car into tight parking spaces because you cannot turn and twist your back and neck to look behind you.
- Special wide-view mirrors fitted to the car can be very helpful. Have some practice sessions driving and backing up the car in an open area to become comfortable using these mirrors. A small hand mirror may be of use in special situations in

avoiding 'blind spot'.

- Use seat belts and head restraints so that sudden slowing or stoppage does not jerk the spine, including the neck. Remember that the stiff neck of an AS patient is more vulnerable to injury than a normal neck. The top of the car seat's head restraint should be level with the top of the your head, and the restraint should be adjustable and as close to the back of your head as possible.
- Avoid bucket seats.
- A disabled driver parking permit may be appropriate for anyone who can't walk very far, but this is usually not a problem for most people with AS.
- If you have a painful and stiff spine, and have difficulty driving a long distance, stop after an hour or two at some appropriate place, and get out of the car to stretch your back and walk around for a few minutes.
- The Ankylosing Spondylitis International Federation (ASIF) has published a booklet for drivers with AS. See Appendix 1 for contact details.

Impact of AS on employment and earning capacity

- Most people with AS are able to cope well, continuing a very productive and active lifestyle.
- Your employer's tolerance for a flexible work schedule or a working environment adapted to your needs can have a great impact on whether or not you are able to get or keep a job. Read the chapter 'Staying employed' in the book *Straight talk on spondylitis* for more information.

- It may be helpful to alter your positions at work, e.g. use short rest periods to perform back stretching exercises during work hours, especially if your work involves prolonged sitting or standing. This can be arranged on consultation with the employer.
- Avoid prolonged stooping and heavy lifting; the work surface should be at a proper height to avoid bending.
- If your current job involves excessive strain on the back because you have to work in a cramped or bent position, you may have to think of a change of job. Vocational rehabilitation agencies are available to provide guidance.
- In a Norwegian disease outcome study of 100 people with adult onset AS, just over half were employed in full-time work after a mean disease duration of 16 years. Stopping work was associated with low levels of education, female sex, recurrent acute iritis, bamboo spine, and the presence of other concommitant non-rheumatic diseases. After more than 20 years of disease, more than 80% of the people surveyed still complained of daily pain and stiffness, and more than 60% needed to take their anti-rheumatic medications daily.
- In the past some people with AS used to get so stooped that they could not even look straight ahead. Some forward stooping of the neck and curvature in the upper back is still commonly observed after many years of the disease. Looking physically different from the rest of the population can present psychological problem, but most people are able to come to terms with this.

- Severe disease that results in complete spinal fusion in bent position and severe limitation of chest expansion, especially when there is also con-tracture of the hip or shoulder joints, may shorten life span because the function of the heart and lungs may be adversely affected and there is a greater risk of spinal fractures.

Health-related quality of life

- Health-related quality of life is based on your perception of the net effects an illness has on your life. It is commonly based on your symp-toms, physical functioning and ability to work, psychosocial functioning and interaction, un-toward effects of treatment, and direct and indirect medical and financial costs.
- Although people with AS are troubled with pain, stiffness, and limited spinal mobility, most of them remain in employment. A recent study at a rheumatology referral center in Germany indi-cates that people with AS have a degree of pain, disability, and reduction in well-being similar to patients with rheumatoid arthritis, a more severe type of arthritis. However, such referral centers are likely to see patients with more severe disease, so their results many not apply to every-one with AS.
- In a recent survey of 175 AS patients (68% male, mean disease duration of 23.7 years, mean age 51 years) the most common quality of life concerns were about stiffness (90%), pain (83%), fatigue (62%), poor sleep (54%), appear-ance (51%), side-effects of medications (41%), and concern about the future (50%). Few

patients in this survey reported problems with social relations or mood.

- There are many recently published journal articles on employment, disability and quality of life of patients with AS. See 'References and further reading section.

Depression

Depression is not uncommon in people with any chronic painful illness that impairs quality of life, and that includes AS. Depression is a treatable disease that has many underlying causes, and some individuals are genetically prone to it. Symptoms of depression include:

- loss of pleasure in activities that were once enjoyable
- persistent feeling of sadness, emptiness, decreased energy, tiredness, and anxiety
- frequently feeling helpless, worthless, guilty, and hopeless, or feeling irritable and restless
- disturbed appetite (loss of appetite or tendency to overeat)
- disturbed sleep (difficulty sleeping, waking up too early, oversleeping, sleeping too little or too much)
- difficulty in concentrating, thinking, remembering, or decision-making
- sometimes persistent physical problems (e.g. headache, abdominal pain) not responding to treatment
- thoughts of ending life by committing suicide.

If you have any of these symptoms you should discuss them with your doctor so that appropriate treatment can be provided.

Additional information on depression is available from the National Institute of Mental Health (*www.nimh.nih.gov*) or the American Psychiatric Association (*www.psych.org*).

12
The management of AS: an overview

- There is currently no preventive measure or a curative treatment for AS, but in most people the disease can be very well managed. Early and more precise diagnosis leads to earlier and more rational or effective therapeutic interventions.
- Splints, braces, and corsets are generally not helpful and are not advised.
- There is no special diet, and there is no evidence that any specific food has anything to do with triggering or increasing the severity of AS.
- Fertility, pregnancy, and childbirth are usually normal in women suffering from AS.
- NSAIDs are very effective in relieving pain and stiffness in most (80%) of the patients with AS. They should be used regularly and in the full therapeutic anti-inflammatory doses during the active phase of the disease. Patients should be made aware of this, since otherwise they may use the NSAIDs only occasionally, for their pain-relieving effect.
- The individual responses to the various NSAIDs may vary from one person to another, as do the

side-effects, so it is worthwhile searching out the best NSAID for each individual.

- When the disease is not adequately controlled by NSAIDS, or for people who are intolerant of such drugs, other medications may be needed, especially in those with peripheral arthritis, inflammatory bowel disease, or psoriasis.
- Newer drugs that neutralize a factor in the body called TNF are very effective, but as yet their long-term side-effects are unknown.
- Oral corticosteroids (cortisone) have no beneficial effect in the long-term management of AS because of serious side-effects, and they do not halt progression of the disease. Persistent joint inflammation may sometimes respond quite well to a local corticosteroid injection.
- Regular exercise is of fundamental importance in preventing or minimizing ankylosis (stiffness) and deformity. Spinal extension exercises and deep breathing exercises should be done routinely once or twice daily.
- Smoking should be avoided.
- People with AS should walk erect, keeping the spine as straight as possible, and sleep on a firm mattress using a thin pillow, just thick enough to allow a horizontal position of the face to prevent pain from overextension of the neck.
- Physical activity that places prolonged strain on back muscles, such as prolonged stooping or bending, should be avoided.
- Formal physiotherapy is of value for learning the proper posture, appropriating exercises and recreational sports, and maintaining the exercise program. Group exercise sessions that include

warm water exercises (hydrotherapy) are very helpful.

- Regular free-style swimming is considered to be one of the best exercises for people with AS.
- People with limited spinal mobility due to AS should avoid manipulation of their back or neck by chiropractors or masseurs because this can be dangerous for anyone with diminished spinal mobility. Such treatments are known to have inadvertently led to spinal fractures.
- People with AS may have difficulty driving a car because of impaired neck mobility, and may find special wide-view mirrors helpful.
- There are many AS self-help and support groups that enlist enthusiastic patient co-operation, provide information about the disease and advice about life and health insurance, jobs, working environment, wide-view mirrors and other useful items (see Appendix 1 for contact details).
- Total hip joint replacement (arthroplasty) gives very good results, and prevents partial or total disability from severe hip disease. Vertebral wedge bone resection may be needed to correct the severe stooping deformity that may occasionally occur, although this surgery carries a relatively high risk of paraplegia. Heart complications may require pacemaker implantation or aortic valve replacement.
- Radiation treatment of the spine has no role in the modern management of AS.

13
The rheumatologist's role

Who is a rheumatologist?

Rheumatologists are physicians uniquely educated and trained to diagnose and treat arthritis and other diseases of the joints, muscles and bones, such as AS and related diseases. In the US, a rheumatologist is a board-certified internist (internal medicine specialist) or pediatrician who has had an additional 2–3 years of specialized rheumatology training. Most of these physicians become certified in rheumatology after passing another board certification examination.

Board-certified rheumatologists are therefore highly trained specialists in diagnosing and treating arthritis and other rheumatic diseases. Many rheumatologists based in academic or hospital rheumatology units help to train other doctors and allied health professionals, as well as providing patient care. They are also involved in conducting clinical and basic scientific research to enhance our understanding and management of rheumatic diseases. Most rheumatologists, however, are in private practice, and some of them have clinical affiliations with academic medical centers.

Interdisciplinary co-operation

The well-established rheumatology units or centers include not only rheumatologists, but also highly trained allied health professionals such as specialist nurses, physiotherapists, occupational therapists, and medical social workers. The rheumatologists work closely with other health professionals such as orthopedists and physiatrists, podiatrists, psychiatrists, psychologists, and dieticians.

The rheumatologist's most important role is to decide on the diagnosis and recommend the right kind of management for your disease. For those reasons a rheumatologist will ask about your detailed medical history and then carry out a clinical examination, sometimes ordering blood tests and X-rays in order to decide how best to treat you. The doctor should also explain the illness and its long-term impact, and an appropriate treatment plan for the future.

You should not be afraid to ask any questions and to ask for any pamphlets, leaflets or other information to help you gain better insight into your disease. Do not hesitate to bring someone with you to the rheumatologist's office if you prefer.

The people with AS most likely to follow a regular exercise program are those who attend a rheumatologist, believe that the exercise is of benefit, and are well motivated and educated.

Consistency rather than quantity of exercise is of utmost importance. It is the doctor's job to relieve your pain and stiffness, and your job to perform regular exercises and to maintain a reasonably good posture. You should see your doctor for periodic follow-up appointments in order to maintain good health.

Many patients with AS may need to be seen by a rheumatologist over an extended period of time, rather than being cared for by their primary care doctor (general practitioner).

If you are unhappy with or have doubts about your treatment, it is quite appropriate to ask for a second opinion from another consultant.

14
Radiology and diagnosis

Radiology

Conventional X-ray is generally quite helpful in diagnosing AS and distinguishing it from other diseases (differential diagnosis); the sacroiliac joints in people who do not have AS will either be normal or show only some degenerative changes, but no erosions typical of sacroiliitis will be present.

The clinical diagnosis of sacroiliitis, however, may be difficult, especially in the early stages, because the sacroiliac joints are deep and virtually motionless, and there may be no obvious tenderness on direct pressure over the joint. A presumptive diagnosis of AS can be confirmed by finding the characteristic changes of AS on an X-ray, because inflammatory involvement and resultant damage of the sacroiliac joint is usually present by the time you seek medical attention. Finding bone erosions, narrowing or fusion of the sacroiliac joints on an X-ray confirms the presence of the disease. Radiographic (X-ray) evidence of sacroiliitis is required for definitive diagnosis, and is the most consistent finding. Radiography can also detect progressive bony fusion of the spine in later stages of the disease.

Because the onset of the disease is usually preceded by a long latent period and a diagnosis is needed to ensure proper and timely treatment, safe and relatively cheap techniques are needed to detect sacroiliitis with a high degree of sensitivity and specificity. A simple anterior–posterior X-ray ('AP view') of the pelvis is usually sufficient for detection of sacroiliitis. However, such an X-ray can sometimes be normal or show only equivocal (unclear) changes in very early stages of the disease (when the structural changes in the joint are still mostly limited to the joint lining (synovial membrane) and the cartilage). In this situation, a magnetic resonance imaging (MRI) scan, possibly enhanced by the injection of a chemical called gadolinium, appears to be the method of choice for the early detection of sacroiliitis.

MRI can also be used for early detection of inflammation (enthesitis) at other sites, because it can show the early changes in cartilage and the underlying bone. Moreover, unlike X-rays, MRI uses no ionizing radiation and is therefore a useful tool, especially in young people, but it is very costly.

The use of MRI has led to a decreasing use of another radiographic imaging method called computed tomography (CT) to detect sacroiliitis. CT provides a better but costlier detailing of bone and joint changes than a conventional X-ray, and is not commonly needed in the diagnosis of AS. Moreover, there is greater radiation exposure from CT than conventional X-ray of the pelvis.

Laboratory findings

Laboratory tests may not be of much help, and there is no single blood test that can specifically diagnose AS, i.e. there is no diagnostic or confirmatory test. However, some blood tests may contribute to the diagnosis of the disease, or correlate with its severity or clinical presentation.

A simple but non-specific blood test called an ESR (erythrocyte sedimentation rate) is one of the indicators of inflammation. This test may help to detect the presence of severe inflammation, and may be of some use in determining, for example, whether the back pain is the result of inflammation or is the more common mechanical or nonspecific type of back pain or strain. However, less than 70% of people with AS have a raised ESR value, even when there is active inflammation. Moreover, this test is influenced by a variety of other factors, such as anemia, age, body weight, pregnancy, and the sex of the individual tested. In a normal young man the ESR is usually less than 20 mm. Another test of inflammation is called CRP (C-reactive protein); this is less likely to be influenced by extraneous factors.

There is no association with a blood test called **rheumatoid factor** (associated with rheumatoid arthritis) or **antinuclear antibodies** (associated with lupus). Therefore, AS and related spondylo-arthropathies are sometimes listed under the term **seronegative spondyloarthritis**.

Laboratory analysis of the joint (synovial) fluid obtained by joint aspiration (arthrocentesis) or biopsy (obtained by a needle or by arthroscopy via an instrument called arthroscope) does not markedly distinguish AS from other inflammatory rheumatic diseases.

The possible use of HLA-B27 as an aid to diagnosis is discussed in Chapter 16.

New York criteria

The current criteria for the diagnosis of AS, known as the modified New York criteria, are shown in Table 2.

Table 2 The generally accepted criteria for AS (modified New York criteria)

1	Low back pain of at least 3 month's duration improved by exercise and not relieved by rest
2	Limitation of lumbar spinal motion in sagittal (sideways) and frontal (forward and backward) planes
3	Chest expansion decreased relative to normal values for the same sex and age
4	Bilateral sacroiliitis grade 2–4 or unilateral sacroiliitis grade 3 or 4

Definite AS if criterion 4 and any one of the other criteria is fulfilled.
Note: These are classification criteria used for case definition and are primarily designed for research purposes.

Other causes of back pain

There are many possible cause of back pain, but by far the most common is mechanical deterioration of the spine. This can take many forms, but is often related to the intervertebral discs. In childhood the central part of these discs consists of over 85% water; there is a slow but steady decrease with aging, down to about 60% by the age of 80 years. As a result the volume of the disc decreases, leading to narrowing of the disc space, causing buckling of the surrounding ligaments (annulus fibrosus and spinal ligaments), and formation of a bony spur (**osteophyte**) at the edges of the spinal vertebral bodies. Clinical back pain related to disc degeneration increases with age, and is accelerated by mechanical stress.

Ankylosing hyperostosis, also called **Forestier's disease** or **diffuse idiopathic skeletal hyperostosis** (DISH), can cause excessive new bone formation along the spine and some other sites. This can result in a stiff spine that may be confused with AS. Other diseases that may be confused with AS include **osteitis condensans ilii**, **Paget's disease** (of the pelvis and spine), and **Scheuermann's disease**. The spread of cancer to the pelvis and the spine, as well as some chronic spinal infections, can also present as back pain.

A bone-thinning disorder called **osteomalacia**, which results from dietary deficiency of vitamin D and lack of adequate skin exposure to sunlight, or may be a result of chronic kidney failure, can cause back pain and may be mistaken for AS or related spondyloarthropathies. **Osteoporosis** can also cause back pain.

Another illness that can cause confusion is a very rare disease of unknown cause, known as **SAPHO syndrome** (because of its salient features: **s**ynovitis, **a**cne, **p**almoplantar pustulosis, **h**yperostosis, and aseptic **o**steomyelitis). This disease causes bone damage that sometimes affects the sacroiliac joints or the spine.

15

The disease process

What happens in AS?

As explained in Chapter 3, the disease usually begins as an inflammation in the sacroiliac joints. When these joints become inflamed they cause pain that you can feel not just over the joints but diffusely over the buttock (gluteal) area. The sacroiliac joints usually become tender on direct firm pressure in the early stages, but the pain and tenderness gradually get less over the years as the sacroiliac joints become fused and replaced by bone. When the inflammation spreads to involve the lumbar spine, you will be aware of low back pain and stiffness.

The inflammation and pain can result in muscle spasm and tenderness, as well as stiffness of the back. There is a natural tendency to stoop forward to minimize the symptoms, because backward stretching is uncomfortable. This can gradually lead to irreversible bad posture, because if the inflammation is not resolved the body begins a gradual repair process that results in further limitation of back motion due to

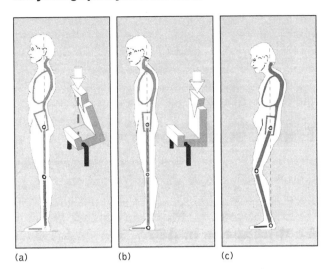

(a)   (b)   (c)

Figure 17 The effects of AS on posture: (a) A healthy person standing erect: Note the hollow lower (lumbar) back and the inclination of the pelvis. Also shown, in a schematic drawing (slightly exaggerated), the transmission of body weight vertically downward (arrow) through the hip joints (black), oblique to the plane of the pelvis. The center of gravity is vertically in line with the hip, knee and ankle joints. (b) A person with a moderately advance stage of AS. Note the upright position of the pelvis and elimination of the lumbar hollow (i.e. straightening of the lower back). The whole static equilibrium is changed; there is some forward stooping of the neck, and the beginnings of upper thoracic kyphosis. (c) A person with very advanced AS, with increased upper thoracic kyphosis and fixed forward stooping of the neck. Note the flexion contracture of the hip joints and the flexed knees, to keep the gaze horizontal. Chest expansion is limited, so the diaphragm must be used for breathing, which makes the abdomen look more prominent ('rubber ball belly'). © Detlef Becker-Capellar.

scarring (fibrous tissue formation) and bone remodelling (Figure 17a, b, c).

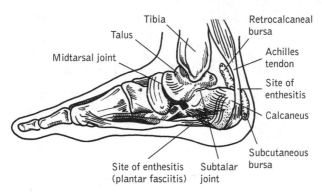

Figure 18

Enthesitis

The inflammation in AS tends to start at the places where joint capsules, ligaments or tendons are attached to bone, resulting in pain or tenderness at these sites. The name **enthesis** is given to these sites, and the inflammatory lesion is called **enthesitis** or sometimes **enthesopathy**.

The doctor should check for pain and tenderness along the back, pelvic bones, sacroiliac joints, and the chest, looking for the presence of enthesitis. There may be heel swelling and tenderness either at the site of insertion of the Achilles tendon to the calcaneus (heel bone), or at the site of the attachment of the plantar fascia to the same bone at the bottom of the heel (see Figure 18). The medical names for these conditions are **Achilles tendinitis**, and **plantar fasciitis** respectively.

A process of healing and repair, which follows the enthesitis phase, results in gradual limitation of back motion due to scarring and subsequent bone

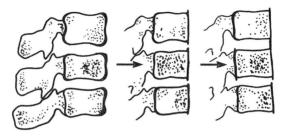

Figure 19

formation. This process may, after many years, lead ultimately to complete spinal fusion. Any clinical examination to look for the presence of AS must therefore include a thorough examination of spinal mobility in all directions (Figure 5), Chapter 3.

The inflammatory changes affect the superficial layers of the ligament (**annulus fibrosus**) that surrounds the disc, especially at its attachment to the corners of the vertebral bodies, resulting in increased bone density (**sclerosis**) of these corners, seen on X-ray as shiny corners (Figure 19). The bone at these corners may subsequently disappear, and this may ultimately result in squaring of the vertebral bodies. Gradually a thin layer of vertical bony outgrowths at the edges of the vertebrae bridges the gap between the two adjacent vertebral bodies, replacing the superficial layer of the annulus fibrosus of the disc. This intervertebral bony bridging that surrounds the disc is called a **syndesmophyte** (Figure 19).

At the same time, inflammatory changes and slowly progressive bony fusion may be going on in spinal joints called the **apophyseal** or **facet joints** (Figure 19). Thus in someone with severe disease the inflammatory process of the spine may gradually, after many years, result in complete fusion (also called **bony ankylosis**) of the whole spine. The X-ray of the spine may ultimately look like a bamboo and is sometimes called **bamboo spine**. Spinal osteoporosis (discussed earlier) is also frequently observed among such patients, partly as a result of the lack of spinal mobility and aging.

The inflammation of the joints between the ribs and the spine (the costovertebral and costotransverse joints), and at the junction of the ribs to the breastbone in front of the chest (the costochondral areas), can result in chest pain and tenderness. This pain can be accentuated by coughing or sneezing. Over the years there may be a gradual decrease in chest expansion. Therefore, some people may present to the doctor with chest pain and tenderness, or complain of inability to expand their chest fully on deep inhalation, or shortness of breath on exertion. The doctor should check not only for limitation of mobility (in all directions) of the spine, including the neck, but also for any restriction of chest expansion (Figure 5f).

Involvement of non-spinal (limb) joints

The hip and shoulder joints, the so-called **girdle joints**, are affected in one-third of AS patients. The hip joint involvement usually affects both sides (bilateral) and is gradual in onset; the pain is usually felt in the groin, although you may feel it in the knee or the front of the thigh on the same side. The hip joint involvement is more common in childhood or adolescence (juvenile AS) when the disease starts. Involvement of the shoulder joint is generally relatively mild.

There is a gradually destruction and thinning of the joint cartilage that cushions the bones of the joints, and this is accompanied by gradual limitation of joint motion. This can give rise to a characteristic rigid gait, with the patient keeping the knees a little bent in an attempt to maintain an erect posture.

In later stages of AS some contracture of the hip joints is not uncommon. For someone whose spine, including the neck, is rigid, involvement of the hips joints is more crippling and can lead to greater disability, but total hip joint replacement can minimize those limitations.

Involvement of peripheral joints, other than hips and shoulders, is quite infrequent except in AS patients who have associated disease, as discussed later. Moreover, such an involvement is rarely persistent or destructive, and usually tends to resolve without any residual joint deformity. Episodes of inflammation of the jaw joint (**temporo-mandibular joint**), occur in about 10% of patients, and cause pain, tenderness, or some limitation in fully opening the mouth.

Involvement of other structures

Spondylitis can also affect structures adjacent to the joints, such as tendons (thick cords that attach muscles to bone) and **bursae** (small sacs between bony prominences and the overlying moving structures such as skin, muscles, or tendons). Inflammation of these structures results in **tendinitis** and **bursitis**.

Some patients complain of fatigue and getting tired easily. There may be wasting (atrophy) and

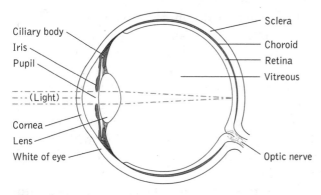

Figure 20

weakness of thigh and buttock muscles due to their
lack of use, especially people with advanced hip
joint involvement. Many such patients have difficulty standing up from a squatting position, and
may need to hold on to something in order to get
up.

Eye inflammation

One or more episodes of acute (abrupt) inflammation of the eye can occur in one-third of all AS
patients at some time in the course of their disease.
This is called acute iritis or anterior uveitis. **Iritis** is
an inflammation of the iris, the colored part of the
eye that surrounds the pupil, and **anterior uveitis**
means inflammation of the iris as well as the adjacent inner layers of the eye (ciliary body) used for
controlling the function of the lens (Figure 20).

Acute iritis may occur before the onset of AS
or even when the disease is otherwise in apparent remission. It usually presents as pain,
redness, difficulty looking directly at bright light,

and excessive tearing in the involved eye. There can be recurrent episodes of acute iritis, but each such episode typically affects one eye only. There may also be some blurring or impairment of vision due to a build-up of inflammatory cells in the front part of the eye. If it is left untreated iritis may have permanent effects on your eyesight, so it requires prompt consultation with an eye specialist (ophthalmologist) for diagnosis and treatment.

Acute iritis can usually be easily managed with dilatation of the pupil and use of corticosteroid eye drops for a few weeks. You may need to use dark glasses temporarily to decrease your sensitivity to bright light. Occasionally, systemic corticosteroids (orally or by injection) or other drugs such as TNF blocking drugs or immunosuppressives may be needed for a few people with severe iritis that has not responded adequately to conventional treatment.

Other associated problems

People with AS should be carefully evaluated for any bowel inflammation, and heart, lung, or neurologic complications. Studies have disclosed the presence of **chronic inflammatory bowel disease**, such as ulcerative colitis and Crohn's disease, in a large number of AS patients, some of whom may have minimal or no bowel symptoms.

In 2–5% of people with AS, usually after many years of the disease, there may be heart involvement in the form of inflammation and scarring. This can affect the heart's electric conduction system, and lead to slowing of the heart rate (**heart block**); or scarring and dilatation of the aorta (the major artery), as it comes out of the heart, and of its valve, may result in a leaky aortic valve (**aortic valve incompetence**). The trouble may, in some patients, be serious enough to require a pacemaker or an aortic valve replacement. Impaired relaxation of the heart muscle, without affecting its ability to contract to pump the blood out, may also be seen in some people with AS.

People with AS who have no symptoms of lung disease do nevertheless get functional lung impairment (documented by **lung function testing**) because of restricted chest expansion. Therefore, some of them may take longer to recover from severe influenza, bronchitis or pneumonia. You should avoid smoking, and discuss with your doctor about the possible need for vaccines against influenza or pneumonia. Scarring (fibrosis) of the upper part (apex) of the lung (**apical fibrosis**) is a rare complication.

16

HLA-B27 and the cause of ankylosing spondylitis

We do not yet know the precise cause of AS, or what triggers it. Along with the other spondylarthropathies, it shows a strong association with a gene called HLA-B27. The disease is most likely caused by multiple predisposing factors, including genetic and non-genetic (environmental) factors. Infections are suspected to be possible environmental triggers. AS may be triggered by gut infection with *Klebsiella* bacteria, but the evidence is circumstantial, and more convincing proof is needed. Some of the other spondylarthropathies, particularly reactive arthritis (Reiter's syndrome), can be triggered after an episode of bowel infection by bacteria, or by infections of the genitourinary tract.

There is substantial evidence that HLA-B27 has a direct role in enhancing genetic susceptibility to AS. However, having the HLA-B27 gene is not a prerequisite for AS, and people without HLA-B27 can also get the disease. Additional genetic factors may influence disease susceptibility, expression or severity; for instance, genes that are suspected to cause susceptibility to psoriasis, ulcerative colitis and Crohn's disease, and possibly other genes yet to be discovered. AS patients have an increased frequency of mild gut inflammation, even though they have no intestinal symptoms or any clinically obvious inflammatory bowel disease (IBD). Follow-up studies of such patients indicate that a small percentage of them will develop clinically obvious Crohn's disease. This suggests that these patients had a sub-clinical form of IBD when they first presented with AS. The presence of this gut inflammation does not show any association with HLA-B27. These findings support the existence of a common link between gut inflammation and AS, independent of HLA-B27. Similar findings have also been observed in patients with other spondyloarthropathies.

What is HLA-B27?

HLA stands for human leucocyte antigens. These are cell surface proteins that vary from person to person. Their function is to help the body fight illness by presenting **peptides** (a few amino acids linked together) derived from foreign proteins (e.g. viral or bacterial), or from the body's own proteins, to T lymphocytes and other cells of the immune system. HLA are the products of genes located on chromosome number 6; the loci (where the genes are located) are given the letters A, B, C, D, and so on.

The HLA genes and their products, i.e. the HLA molecules, are grouped into two broad classes called HLA class I and class II. HLA-B27, or simply B27 for short, is so called because its gene is located at the B locus belonging to the HLA class I group and is assigned the number 27. Many varieties of these genes at these various loci exist in the general population, so it is very difficult to find two unrelated individuals possessing an exactly identical combination of these variations. Any cell that is infected, e.g. by a virus, will usually display on its surface peptide antigens of viral origin, in addition to self-antigens, in combination with HLA class I molecules, such as HLA-B27. The presence of the viral peptide antigens with the HLA molecule activates CD8+ **cytotoxic T cells** specific for that peptide antigen to destroy the infected cell.

The role of HLA-B27 in disease predisposition

A greater prevalence of AS is observed in HLA-B27-positive first-degree relatives of AS patients than in HLA-B27-positive random controls. This suggests that AS is probably genetically heterogeneous, i.e. there are other genetic predisposing factors as well as HLA-B27. However, the evidence favors the gene for HLA-B27 being the major genetic susceptibility factor responsible for AS. The more disease-predisposing genes you inherit the more likely you are to suffer from AS, but most likely it still requires some, as yet unknown, environmental (i.e. non-genetic) trigger for the disease to start.

Although people who are born with the HLA-B27 gene are more predisposed to AS or one of the related spondyloarthropathies (i.e. they are more likely to suffer from these diseases), most of them remain unaffected. It is important to emphasize that there are far more people in the general population with HLA-B27 who never get AS than those who do. Even in families where one member has the disease and the HLA-B27 gene, most of their brothers and sisters will remain unaffected even when they have the same gene.

Perhaps the HLA-B27-positive person destined to develop spondyloarthropathy may be exposed to certain gut organisms that partially imitate HLA-B27 in ways that lead the bacterial antigens to become immunogenic and somehow trigger the disease. The HLA-B27 protein itself or the peptide bound to and derived from HLA-B27 may have a pathogenic role.

Inheritance of HLA-B27

Each of us has 46 chromosomes in the nucleus of our cells, and each chromosome is a tiny thread-like structure that contains a set of genes. We derive 23 of our chromosomes from one parent and the other 23 from the other parent. **Autosomes** is the name given to the 22 of these pairs of chromosomes that are unrelated to the sex of the person; they are assigned numbers 1 through 22, based on their size. The remaining two chromosomes are assigned the letters X and Y, and they are the **sex chromosomes**. Each female has two X chromosomes and each male has an X and a Y chromosome. The father contributes a set of 22 autosomes and an X or a Y chromosome to the offspring, while the mother contributes the other set of 22 autosomes and the X chromosome.

Everyone has two HLA-B genes (one on each chromosome 6), and someone is said to be HLA-B27 positive if B27 is the gene present at either one or both of these HLA-B gene locations.

- If an individual has inherited B27 from both parents so that the B27 gene is present at both of the HLA-B gene location (**B27 homozygous**) then all of that person's children will inherit B27.

- If one parent has HLA-B27 at one of these HLA-B gene locations, as is the case for 8% of people of Western European extraction, then there is a 1 in 2 chance that their offspring will inherit this gene.

- The likelihood of both parents possessing the HLA-B27 gene is less than 7 per 1000. There is then a 1 in 4 chance that the offspring from such a marriage will inherit B27 from both parents (B27 homozygous), a 1 in 2 chance of inheriting the B27 gene from only one parent (**B27 heterozygous**), and a 1 in 4 chance of not inheriting the B27 gene at all.

Genetic counseling

Because of this genetic predisposition, it is not unusual for more than one person in a family to be affected with AS or related diseases, and it is helpful for the doctor to know this family history. A person with AS (who has a >90% chance of possessing the HLA-B27 gene if he or she is of Western European extraction) may ask, *'What is the risk of my children developing it, and can anything be done to prevent this?'*

Children who inherit HLA-B27 from the B27-positive parent with AS (and on average 50% will inherit the B27 gene) carry a risk of up to 1 in 4 of developing the disease themselves during their lifetime.

Thus, most children with the B27 gene do not develop the disease, and the 50% of children who lack the gene carry no virtually increased risk unless genes for other diseases that also predispose to AS (such as psoriasis and inflammatory bowel disease) are present in the family.

If the person with AS does not possess HLA-B27 (a <10% chance if he or she is of Western European extraction), then the risk of disease occurrence among the children may not be increased at all, unless genes for other diseases that also predispose to AS (as mentioned above) are present in the family.

The person with AS, who has a >90% chance of possessing the HLA-B27 gene, may ask, 'Should I have all my children tested for the HLA-B27?' The answer is no, because among the 50% of the children who are expected to be positive, an overwhelming majority (>80%) remain unaffected during their lifetime. Moreoever, the parents and the healthcare providers may get 'HLA-B27-itis': knowing that the child has HLA-B27, the parents and the healthcare providers can worry unnecessarily; and symptoms unrelated to AS may be wrongly attributed to the fact that the child has inherited the gene. Thus the child may get a wrong diagnostic label of AS, even though he or she is an unaffected individual who happens to possess a normal gene called HLA-B27. Even a child who remains totally healthy may suffer indirectly in future if the information about the HLA-B27 test result enters their medical records, and thus becomes available to health insurance agencies, or future potential employers, who may misuse such information.

If a child of an AS parent develops symptoms or signs that you suspect may be due to AS or another HLA-B27 associated disease, you should point out all the child's symptoms to their doctor, who should preferably be a pediatric rheumatologist. When it is appropriate the doctor can utilize HLA-B27 typing as an aid to diagnosis.

HLA-B27 testing in disease diagnosis

AS can almost always be readily diagnosed on the basis of history, physical examination and X-ray findings, and therefore HLA-B27 typing is not necessary for disease diagnosis. A knowledge of the presence of HLA-B27 can sometimes be valuable as an aid to diagnosis, although the prevalence of HLA-B27 (Table 3) and the strength of its association with AS vary markedly in different ethnic and racial groups. For example, only 50% of African– American patients with AS possess HLA-B27, and it is close to 80% among AS patients from Mediterranean countries.

Thus, AS and related diseases can also occur in people who do not have HLA-B27. Therefore, a negative test result for B27 does not, in itself, completely exclude the presence of the disease. Moreover, a positive test result in itself does not mean that someone has the disease, because the HLA-B27 gene is present in a significant percentage of the healthy general population.

However, the test can be useful for a doctor who understands the principles of probability reasoning and uses it only in a toss-up clinical situation. In other words, the doctor may think that there is a 40–60% likelihood that the patient has AS, and the sacroiliac joint X-rays are either normal or show equivocal (not very definite) changes. Moreover, its clinical usefulness is influenced by the patient's racial and ethnic background. Typing for HLA-B27 should not be considered a routine, diagnostic, confirmatory, or screening test for AS in patients with back pain in the general population.

Research on HLA-B27 and related topics

Prevalence of HLA-B27 in world populations

HLA-B27 is not uncommon in the general population, but its prevalence varies among different ethnic/racial groups throughout the world. This is shown in Table 3. The numbers are rounded off for simplicity, and indicate percentage prevalence in the general population. For example, in the USA approximately 8% of whites and 2–3% of African-Americans posses this gene, but it is much more common among the native Americans.

In general, AS and related diseases are more common in populations with a relatively higher prevalence of HLA-B27, such as among the Inuit and Eskimos, and the converse is also true (Table 4). HLA-B27 and AS are both absent from Australian aboriginal populations of unmixed genetic ancestry. However, there are some exceptions to this generalization; e.g. AS is virtually absent in certain West African populations even though HLA-B27 is present in up to 6% of them.

Different types of HLA-B27

So far, 25 different types of HLA-B27 (named B*2701 to B*2725) have been distinguished; most of them are quite rare. The presence of the different HLA-B27 subtypes also differs markedly among the

Table 3 Percentage prevalence of HLA-B27 in different populations throughout the world.

Native American linguistic population groups		
Eskimo-Aleut	Eskimos and Inuit	25–40
Na-Dene	Tlingit, Dogrib, and Navajo	20–35
Amerind	Bella co-ola	26
	Yakima and Pima	18–21
	Cree, Zuni and Chippewa	11–14
	Papago, Hopi and Havasupai	7–9
	Mexican Mestizo	3–6
	Central American natives	4–20
	South American natives	0
North and central Asiatic linguistic population groups		
Chukchic	Siberian Chuckchis	19–34
	Siberian Eskimo	40
Uralic	Ural mountain natives	8–15
	Samis (Lapps)	24
Altaic	Siberians: Yakuts	17–19
	Tofs	13
	Buryats	3–6
	Japanese	1
	Ainu (native Japanese)	4
	Koreans, Uygurs and Mongolians	3–9
	Uzbeks, Kazakhs and Turkic populations	3–8
Sino-Tibetan	Chinese (mainland)	2–6
	Chinese (overseas)	4–9
	Tibetans	12
Caucasoid populations	Ugro-Finnish	12–18
	Northern Scandinavians	10–16
	Slavic populations	7–14
	Western Europeans	6–9
	Mediterranean Europeans	2–6
	Basques	9–14
	Gypsies (Spain)	16–18
	Arabs, Jews, Armenians, and Iranians	1–6
	Pakistanis	6–8
	Indians (Asian)	2–6
Other Asiatic populations		
South-east Asians	Vietnamese	9
	Khmer, Taiwanese aborigines and Filipinos	5–8

Table 3 (contd)

	Indonesians, Malaysians and Thais	5–12
Micronesians	Nauru	2
	Guam	5
Melanesians	Papua New Guineans	12–26
	Vanuatuans and New Caledonians	18–23
	Ouveans	11
	Fijians	4–6
Polynesians	Hawaians, Samoans and Marquesas Islanders	2–3
	Maoris	0–3
	Tokelau and Society Islanders	0
	Rapanui (Easter Islanders)	0
	Australian aborigines	0
North and West African populations		
North Africans	Arabs	3–5
	Berbers	2
	Ethiopians	1
West Africans	Gambia and Senegal	2– 6
	Mali	10
Equatorial and Southern African populations		
	Pygmies	7–10
	San (Bushmen)	0
	Bantu	
	Nigerians	0
	Zimbabweans	0
	South African Xhosas	0–0.3
	Zaireans	0–0.7

various world populations. For example, HLA-B*2705 is the most common subtype among white people, and the Siberian and North American native populations, whereas HLA-B*2704 is the most common subtype among the Chinese and Japanese populations, HLA-B*2706 (B*2722) is the most common subtype among Indonesians, and HLA-B*2703 is only observed among West Africans or people with African ancestry.

Table 4 Recent prevalence studies of AS and related spondyloarthropathies

	HLA-B27 frequency in general population (%)	Prevalence of AS (%) in general adult population	in B27-positive adult population	Prevalence of spondyloarthropathies (including AS) in general adult population	in B27-positive adult population
Eskimos (Alaska)	40	0.4		2.5	
Eskimos (Alaska and Siberia and Chukcki)	25–40		1.6	2–3.4	4.2
Samis (Lapps)	24	1.8	6.8		
Northern Norway	10–16	1.4			
Mordovia	16	0.5			
Western Europe	8	0.2			
Germany (Berlin)	9	0.9	6.4	1.9	13.6

Association of different types of HLA-B27 with AS

The presence of AS or related spondyloarthropathies has been noted in individuals born with any of the common HLA-B27 subtypes so far known. However, two subtypes seem to be, at the most, only very weakly associated with disease. These are HLA-B*2722 (formerly mistyped as HLA-B*2706), which is found in south-east Asian populations, and HLA-B*2709, a rare subtype observed in Italian populations, primarily on the island of Sardinia.

Other research studies

If a cell is infected, by a virus for example, it will display on its surface small protein molecules called peptides, of viral or self-origin, in combination with **HLA class I molecules**, such as HLA-B27. The presence of the viral peptide antigens with the HLA molecule activates CD8+ T cells (cytotoxic T cells, which are destructive to cells) which are specific for that antigen. Certain types of HLA are more efficient in defending against certain infections, but at the same time they may make the individual more vulnerable to developing certain other infections or diseases. For example, an individual born with HLA-B27 is able to mount a better response against many viruses (as compared to others born with HLA genes other than HLA-B27), but they are somehow more likely to suffer from AS or related spondyloarthropathies.

HLA class II molecules are found on cells, such as macrophages, which present antigens to the immune system and are therefore called **antigen-presenting cells**. When these cells ingest bacteria or their products, or are infected by bacteria, they display peptide antigens on their surface, including those derived from bacterial proteins and toxins, in combination with HLA class II molecules. CD4+ (helper) T cells specific for these peptide antigens then help mount an immune response against the infection.

Laboratory rats and mice have been raised that carry the human HLA-B27 genes. These so-called HLA-B27 transgenic rats and mice express HLA-B27 on their cell surface. They have been very helpful in finding out how HLA-B27 may predispose humans to AS and related spondyloarthropathies. The HLA-B27 transgenic rats spontaneously develop an inflammatory disease that shares many features with the human spondyloarthropathies, including sacroiliitis. Breeding the animals in a germ-free environment has allowed the disease to be differentiated into those features that require normal bacteria in the gut (i.e. the occurrence of diarrhea followed by arthritis) and those that don't (psoriasis-like skin and nail lesions). The disease is produced by T cells recognizing HLA-B27 expressed at high levels on bone-marrow-derived antigen-presenting cells, and there is a critical requirement for bacterial components.

Family studies

The discovery of the remarkable association of HLA-B27 with AS and related spondyloarthropathies was reported in 1973. It helped to revitalize the clinical and genetic studies of these disorders, and also broadened our understanding of their wider clinical spectrum. However, we still do not know exactly how HLA-B27 plays its role in disease predisposition.

Familial occurrence of these diseases provides a potential clinical resource for uncovering all the genes, other than HLA-B27, that make an individual susceptible to environmental (non-genetic) triggers that start the disease process. However, these environmental triggers are also not yet fully known.

Research studies of families where two or more first-degree relatives suffer from AS are currently taking place in North America and Europe. The study involves obtaining blood samples from members of such families. The DNA from these samples is then analyzed in the research laboratory in order to find all the genes that play a role in disease predisposition. Such genetic studies have not as yet had an impact on clinical medicine, but once we have a greater understanding of how genes interact with the environmental agents that trigger diseases, it will be possible to treat them more effectively and even prevent them.

17
Spondyloarthropathies

The spondyloarthropathies are related diseases that include AS. The various forms of spondyloarthropathy usually begin in the late teens and early twenties, but they can also begin in childhood or later in life. They show a strong association with HLA-B27, but the strength of this association varies markedly, not only between the various spondyloarthropathies but also among racial and ethnic groups.

The mode of presentation of spondyloarthropathies is very varied and, with the exception of AS, may not necessarily involve sacroiliitis or spondylitis. It may also not be always possible to differentiate clearly between the various forms of spondyloarthropathies, especially in their early stages, because they generally share many clinical features, both skeletal and extra-skeletal. However, this is not a serious clinical problem because it does not usually impact the treatment decisions.

Spondyloarthropathies other than AS include:

- the arthritis associated with chronic inflammatory bowel diseases (i.e. ulcerative colitis and Crohn's disease) or psoriasis (a chronic skin disease)

- a form of juvenile chronic arthritis
- reactive arthritis (Reiter's syndrome)
- undifferentiated forms of the disease.

Patients with psoriasis, ulcerative colitis, Crohn's disease, or reactive arthritis (Reiter's syndrome) are more likely to develop AS than the rest of the population. The reverse is also true, i.e. patients with AS are more likely than the general population to also suffer from Crohn's disease, ulcerative colitis, or psoriasis.

Doctors have found that the clinical features typical of spondyloarthropathies may occur in different combinations, so the existing criteria for disease classification may not be appropriate for some patients. The European Spondyloarthropathy Study Group (**ESSG**) have therefore developed classification criteria (Table 5) to include this currently recognised wider spectrum of spondyloarthropathies.

Reactive arthritis (Reiter's syndrome)

Reactive arthritis is an aseptic inflammatory arthritis that follows an episode of urethritis, cervicitis, or diarrhea, and may also show inflammation at sites other than joints, such as eyes, skin, and mouth. The joint inflammation is triggered by bacterial infection at a distant site, usually in the gastrointestinal or genitourinary tract.

Not everyone who develops these bacterial infections will develop reactive arthritis. Some people are genetically susceptible and the inheritance of the HLA-B27 gene increases the risk of

Table 5 The European Spondyloarthropathy Study Group (ESSG) criteria for classifying disease as a spondyloarthropathy

Spondyloarthropathy is defined as the presence of **inflammatory spinal pain** or **synovitis** *and*

one or more of the following:

- **family history:** presence, in first- or second-degree relatives, of: ankylosing spondylitis, psoriasis, acute iritis, reactive arthritis, or inflammatory bowel disease.
- **psoriasis**
- **inflammatory bowel disease**
- **alternating buttock pain**
- **enthesitis**
- **acute diarrhea**
- **urethritis**
- **sacroiliitis:** bilateral grade 2–4 or unilateral grade 3–4

Definitions used in these criteria

Inflammatory spinal pain: history of or current symptoms of spinal pain (low, mid and upper back, or neck region), with at least four of the following five components:

a   at least 3 months duration
b   onset before age 45
c   insidious (gradual) onset
d   improved by exercise
e   associated with morning spinal stiffness

Synovitis: past or present asymmetric arthritis, or arthritis predominately in the lower limbs

Psoriasis: past or present psoriasis diagnosed by a doctor

Inflammatory bowel disease: past or present ulcerative colitis or Crohn's disease diagnosed by a doctor and confirmed by radiographic examination or endoscopy

Alternating buttock pain: past or present pain alternating between the two buttock regions

Enthesitis: past or present spontaneous pain or tenderness at examination of the site of the insertion of the Achilles tendon or plantar fascia

Acute diarrhea: episode of diarrhea occurring within 1 month before arthritis onset

Urethritis: nongonococcal urethritis or cervicitis occurring within 1 month before arthritis onset

Sacroiliitis grading system: 0 = normal, 1 = possible, 2 = minimal, 3 = moderate, 4 = completely fused (ankylosed).

reactive arthritis by about 50-fold. The disease tends to be more severe and more likely to become chronic in people with a triggering infection that is symptomatic and proven by bacterial culture, especially if they are born with the HLA-B27 gene, than if the triggering infection produces no symptoms and is suggested only by a positive antibody test.

Depending on the bacterial trigger, reactive arthritis can be more common in men than in women. Table 6 lists some of the important bacterial triggers. Genitourinary tract infection with *Chlamydia* is the more commonly recognized initiator in the US, but enteric infections with *Shigella, Salmonella, Yersinia,* or *Campylobacter* are more common triggers in developing countries. Sometimes there is no recognized antecedent infection, or the triggering infection may be asymptomatic. The term **reactive arthritis** is often used when the identity of the triggering organism is known, and it encompasses the more restrictive and less commonly used term **Reiter's syndrome.**

Table 6 Bacteria triggering reactive arthritis

Chlamydia trachomatis
Shigella flexneri
Salmonella (many species)
Yersinia enterocolitica and *Y. pseudotuberculosis*
Campylobacter fetus jejuni
Clostridium difficile

Note: Reactive arthritis not associated with HLA-B27 has also been observed following many bacterial, viral and parasitic infections, and in association with intestinal bypass surgery, acne, hidradenitis suppurative (abscesses in the armpit and groin), and cystic fibrosis.

How common is reactive arthritis?

The prevalence of reactive arthritis in a population varies with that of HLA-B27 and the triggering bacterial infections. *Chlamydia*-induced reactive arthritis is most commonly seen in young promiscuous men. However, it is under-diagnosed in women because their chlamydial infection is often subclinical or asymptomatic, and also because doctors rarely do pelvic examinations to look for the presence of cervicitis (inflammation of the cervix, the part of the uterus that protrudes into the vagina). The post-enteritic form of the disease affects children and adults, both male and female, including elderly people.

The incidence of *Chlamydia*-induced reactive arthritis has declined since 1985 in Europe and the US, but the post-enteritic form of the disease may be increasing. After some epidemics of bacterial gastroenteritis or food poisoning (e.g. *Salmonella* enteritis) the incidence of reactive arthritis, or at least some form of musculoskeletal inflammation and pain, can be as high as 20% among B27-positive individuals in the general population, but the initial episode of reactive arthritis in such epidemics is relatively weakly associated with HLA-B27 (not more than 33% of these patients may possess this gene).

To give one specific example, in the Finnish general population aged 18–60 years the annual incidence of *Chlamydia*-induced reactive arthritis (confirmed by bacterial culture) is 4.6 per 100 000. The triggering genitourinary infection is asymptomatic in 36%. The annual incidence of post-enteritic reactive arthritis is 5 per 100 000; the triggering enteric infection is asymptomatic in 26%.

Symptoms of reactive arthritis

The clinical picture varies from mild **arthritis** to a severely disabling illness that may render the patient bedridden for a few weeks. Many people have only one episode, but in some the disease does recur or persist. The arthritis more frequently involves the lower limbs, with the knees and ankles being most commonly affected, followed by the feet, the upper limbs, and the back. General symptoms such as malaise, fever, and aching muscles (myalgia) may occur, and there may also be pain in the lower back and the buttocks that feels worse in the early morning.

The acute arthritis is often associated with conjunctivitis or urethritis. **Conjunctivitis** (commonly known as **pink eye**) is an inflammation of the delicate outer membrane that lines the inside of the eyelids and the white of the eye. The inflammation is usually mild and bilateral, and you may not even notice it. However, it can cause eye irritation and redness, and sometimes your eyelids may stick together in the morning. Some patients may get **acute iritis** (see Chapter 15).

Urethritis, an inflammation of the urethra (a small tube through which urine passes from the bladder to the outside), can cause difficult or painful urination. It occurs much more commonly in post-chlamydial reactive arthritis, and is more frequently symptomatic in men than in women, and may sometimes result in slight pus- or mucus-like urethral discharge, bladder inflammation (cystitis), lower abdomen pain, and urinary frequency. Sometimes the urethritis symptoms may be quite mild, and the doctor will have to ask about them.

Prostatitis (an infection or inflammation of the prostate gland in men) often occurs in conjunction with urethritis. Women may develop cervicitis but often there are no symptoms, and it may only be detected by a pelvic examination.

People with post-enteritic reactive arthritis often describe a history of fever, abdominal pain and diarrhea, preceding the arthritis by 1–4 weeks. They may sometimes also have sterile (non-infected) urethritis.

Skin lesions can cause a lot of anxiety. A skin rash resembling psoriasis may appear on the soles of the feet and palms of the hands. These skin lesions are called **keratoderma blennorrhagica**, and often heal within a few weeks but may need prescription creams. In a few people small, shallow, painless sores may occur on the tongue or roof of the mouth (palate), but they usually heal in a few days or weeks without any scarring, even without any treatment. Similar sores, called **circinate balanitis**, sometimes occur on the external genitalia – on the tip (glans) or shaft of the penis or on the scrotum in men, and in the vagina in women. They crust over and heal after a few weeks. Finger- and/or toe-nails may show nail discoloration similar to that seen in psoriasis, but without nail pitting or ridging.

Enthesitis is an important hallmark of reactive arthritis, and tendon sheaths and bursae may also become inflamed. Sausage-like swelling of the toes or fingers may be a prominent finding in some patients, just as in psoriatic arthritis. In the ankle, enthesitis can cause swelling, pain and tenderness in the back of the foot (**Achilles tendinitis**). Heel pain due to inflammation of the tendons, attached to the heel, which support, the arch of the foot (**plantar fasciitis**) is a frequent complaint. Ligamentous structures along the spine and sacroiliac joints, and around the ankle and mid-foot, may also become inflamed. Psoriatic arthritis shares many features with reactive arthritis, and sometimes a long period of observation may be needed to reach a correct diagnosis.

Diagnosis

Diagnosis may sometimes be difficult, as there is no specific diagnostic test. The erythrocyte sedimentation rate (ESR) is often high, but this is common in inflammatory diseases. Other tests include examination and cultures of synovial (joint) fluid, stool, and urethral discharge. A careful clinical history and physical examination is needed to diagnose this condition. Because there is a delay of several days between the triggering infection and the onset of disease, the patient may not relate the two events and therefore not mention the previous episode of infection to the doctor.

Outcome

In most people the disease can be well-managed with treatment, and the outcome is usually good because the disease is often self-limiting, i.e. it goes away without any residual problems. Other people may have recurrent attacks or have a chronic form of the disease with ongoing joint problems, typically recurring arthritis and tendinitis that may result in stiff joints and weak muscles.

Back and neck pain and stiffness due to sacroiliitis and spondylitis may also occur. X-ray evidence of sacroiliac joint involvement is seen in about 10% of patients during the acute phase, and much more frequently in chronic cases. The spondylitis usually does not lead to the bamboo spine typical of AS.

HLA-B27 is present in up to 70% of people with reactive arthritis, compared to 8% in the general population of Western European descent. The association is weaker among some of the other races (e.g. only up to 40% of African–American reactive arthritis patients, and 2–3% of their general population possess B27). The presence of HLA-B27 can be of some value as an aid to diagnosis in some appropriate clinical situations, but its absence cannot be used to exclude the diagnosis because many people with reactive arthritis do not have HLA-B27. Patients who are B27-positive are more likely to have back pain and stiffness, although sacroiliitis is often not visible on X-ray in early stages. The disease is more likely to become chronic and evolve into spondylitis or be associated with acute iritis in people who are B27-positive.

Psoriatic arthritis

Psoriasis is a very common chronic skin disease, especially in populations of European extraction, and is present in up to 2% of the US population. There is abnormal proliferation of skin cells (called **keratinocytes**), induced by T lymphocytes, but the precise cause is unknown. Psoriasis is usually seen in the form of itchy, dry, red, and scaly patches of skin. Finger- and toenails may show discoloration (**onycholysis**), accompanied by pitting and ridging.

An inflammatory arthritis occurs in more than 10% of people with psoriasis. The arthritis precedes the onset or the diagnosis of psoriasis in approximately 15% of them. A family history of psoriasis or psoriatic arthritis is present in up to 40% of people with psoriatic arthritis, and family studies suggest that several genes are involved (a **multigenic** mode of inheritance). Psoriasis is relatively much less common in African-Americans, native Americans, and south-east Asians. The disease affects men and women equally and usually begins between 30–50 years of age although it can begin in childhood.

Sausage-like diffuse swelling of the toes or fingers ('**sausage digits**') may be a prominent finding in some patients, and enthesitis at bony sites of attachment of ligaments and tendons can cause painful heels and a tender back. X-rays of the affected joints may show anything from mild erosion to severe bone destruction and occasionally fusion of the joints. Psoriatic arthritis has been divided into five types:

- inflammatory arthritis, primarily involving the distal small joints of fingers or toes
- asymmetric inflammatory arthritis, involving a few of the joints of the limbs
- symmetrical arthritis of multiple joints, resembling rheumatoid arthritis
- arthritis mutilans, a rare but very deforming and destructive (mutilating) form
- arthritis of the sacroiliac joint and the spine (psoriatic spondylitis)

The exact prevalence of each of these forms of arthritis is difficult to establish. Disease patterns may differ among various population groups, and may even change with time in an individual. Some patients may show overlapping features. Sacroiliitis occurs in about 15% and predominant spondylitis in about 5%. Some people may get conjunctivitis or acute iritis. Spondylitis and acute iritis are more common in those who are B27-positive.

Enteropathic arthritis

Enteropathic arthritis develops in up to 20% of people with Crohn's disease or ulcerative colitis. This arthritis usually takes the form of peripheral joint inflammation that correlates with flare-up of the bowel disease, especially in the case of ulcerative colitis, but one-fourth have axial disease (sacroiliitis alone or with classic AS) that does not fluctuate with bowel disease activity.

Subclinical inflammatory lesions in the gut have been observed in spondyloarthropathy patients without gut symptoms. Follow-up studies suggest that 15–25% of them will eventually develop clinically obvious Crohn's disease, suggesting that they initially had a subclinical form of this disease.

Childhood (juvenile) spondyloarthropathies

Juvenile spondyloarthropathies are defined as having their onset before the age of 16. Recent data from pediatric rheumatology clinic registries in Canada, the UK, and the US indicate that approximately 8% of all children referred to pediatric rheumatic disease clinics have a spondyloarthropathy, and among those children identified as having a discrete rheumatic disease, approximately 20% suffer from spondyloarthropathy.

Improved guidelines for diagnosing childhood rheumatic diseases have contributed to earlier identification of childhood spondyloarthropathies. There is often no chronic inflammatory lower back pain, sacroiliitis, psoriatic skin lesions, or intestinal symptoms, and as discussed later, undifferentiated forms of spondyloarthropathies occur more often during childhood and adolescence than in adulthood. Many patients may show a family history of AS, psoriasis, inflammatory bowel disease, or acute iritis. These spondyloarthropathies show a strong association with HLA-B27, just like AS of adult onset.

Intermittent episodes of pain in the groin, and resultant limping, without any previous physical trauma or infection, can be a presenting manifestation in some children. Others may present with enthesitis at multiple sites. Some may present with the syndrome of enthesits and arthritis (sometimes called SEA syndrome, which stands for seronegative enthesitis and arthritis). If the enthesitis affects the site of attachment of the patellar tendon to the tibial tubercle (a bony prominence an inch or so below the kneecap), it can sometimes be confused with a childhood condition called **Osgood–Schlatter's disease**. However, a child with juvenile spondyloarthropathy will frequently also show tenderness at other bony sites due to enthesitis, and not just at the tibial tubercles.

At least 50% of these young people reach adulthood with persistent (active) arthritis and need further rheumatological care. Their disease may evolve into juvenile-onset AS with back pain, sacroiliitis, and diminished spinal mobility. A study of such patients in Mexico has found that severe enthesitis in the feet is a very common first presentation of AS in a Mestiso population of mixed genetic ancestry (mostly native Americans with some Spanish admixture).

Reactive arthritis including Reiter's syndrome can also occur in children, usually triggered by enteric infection due to *Shigella*, *Salmonella*, or *Yersinia*. There is an association with HLA-B27, but the arthritis is relatively less severe than in adults. The juvenile onset of psoriatic arthritis is uncommon but well documented.

Undifferentiated spondyloarthropathy

The term 'undifferentiated' is used for a limited form or early stage of the disease that does not meet the criteria for AS, or the other spondyloarthropathies described above, which could be considered as differentiated spondyloarthropathies. The undifferentiated forms can occur in adults too, but are relatively more common in children. In fact, at least 50% of spondyloarthropathies of childhood onset present in an undifferentiated form.

The disease may begin with enthesitis causing pain in the heels and other bony sites, or lower extremity arthritis of one (especially knee or ankle) or more joints, mostly in boys between the ages of 9 and 16 years, without any other features. This form of arthritis may precede the back pain by several years.

Less than 1 in 4 of children with AS or other differentiated spondyloarthropathies initially present with back pain, stiffness, or restricted motion, or symptoms or signs of sacroiliitis. This is a notable distinction from adults with AS. When a young child presents with isolated signs referable to the sacroiliac joint, possible bacterial infection of the sacroiliac joint is also considered. Sometimes leukemia and other forms of malignancy in children may mimic the clinical presentation of juvenile arthritis, including spondyloarthropathy.

X-ray evidence of sacroiliitis is one of the diagnostic hallmarks of spondyloarthropathies in the adult population. However, it is not easy to detect sacroiliitis by conventional radiography in growing children. Dynamic **MRI** is helpful in children and adolescents with clinical features suggestive of a spondyloarthropathy, because it can distinguish normal growth changes from true inflammatory disease, and it does not involve exposure to radiation.

Treatment of spondyloarthropathies other than AS

The initial treatment consists of the use of NSAIDs to treat joint problems. Persistent arthritis or enthesitis may require a corticosteroid injection into the affected area. This is particularly helpful if the pain and swelling continues to persist in one or more joints. If the arthritis does not resolve within a few weeks, additional medications such as sulfasalazine (Salazopyrin) or methotrexate (Rheumatrex) may be needed. Anti-TNF therapy is very effective for patients with juvenile chronic arthritis resistant to conventional therapy.

Daily exercises stretching the joints involved (to keep them from getting stiff), and muscle-strengthening exercises (to regain strength and prevent muscle wasting and weakness) may be needed. Application of local heat or a warm shower may promote relaxation and help in passive stretching of tight muscles. A heated swimming pool may also help to decrease pain. When the acute phase of the arthritis resolves, low-impact exercises in the water (swimming and water aerobics) and stationary exercise bicycling can help improve exercise capability, muscle strength, and range of motion of the affected joint. Surgery can be helpful for people with severe joint damage.

Treatment of skin involvement in psoriatic arthritis

Psoriasis responds to topical corticosteroid medications (ointments and creams), exposure to ultraviolet A light after application of photosensitizing psoralene—the so called psoralen-photo-augmented ultraviolet A (PUVA) treatment, or treatment with vitamin D analogs. It is inadvisable to prescribe corticosteroids by mouth to treat psoriasis because this has untoward effects; in particular, the rapid tapering down of the dose can result in flare-up of skin disease. Refractory skin lesions may need methotrexate or sulfasalazine. **Cyclosporin** has been used with good results, as has **anti-TNF therapy**, however, because of their side-effects and their high cost, these are only suitable for people with progressive disease unresponsive to other measures.

Several studies have demonstrated that antibiotic treatment does not influence the course of reactive arthritis that has been triggered by enteric infection. It seems that once the enteritis trigger has been pulled, the chain of events takes its path anyway. However, vigorous antibiotic treatment of *Chlamydia* re-infections has significantly reduced relapses of reactive arthritis triggered by this organism.

Reactive arthritis itself is not contagious; only the triggering bacteria are. If the preceding infection is transmitted sexually, as is the case with urogenital chlamydial infection, it is advisable for the patient's sexual partners to be treated with antibiotics at the same time. This helps to eradicate the infection, or at least prevent it being transmitted to others.

Use of sulfasalazine or methotrexate in people unresponsive to NSAIDs

Because of the efficacy of sulfasalazine in the treatment of inflammatory bowel disease and psoriasis even in the absence of any associated arthritis, this drug may be especially useful for spondyloarthropathies associated with those diseases.

People with severe spondyloarthropathies with peripheral joint involvement who are unresponsive to NSAIDs and sulfasalazine have sometimes responded to weekly oral methotrexate (Rheumatrex) therapy. Sometimes other immunosuppressants, such as azathioprine (Imuran), have been used in the treatment of chronic inflammatory arthritis resistant to conventional therapy. It is important to remember that sulfasalazine and immunosuppressants are relatively slow-acting anti-rheumatic drugs, so patients should not expect a quick response. Moreover, these drugs, unlike NSAIDs, are not pain relievers, although they can help relieve pain if they can first heal or control the underlying inflammation that contributes to it.

Some patients with inflammatory bowel disease may need corticosteroid enemas or even oral corticosteroids for control of severe flare-up consultations of the bowel disease, and also require regular follow-up consultations with their gastroenterologist. Treatment of severe chronic inflammatory bowel disease, specifically Crohn's disease, with infliximab (Remicade), is very effective, and may also control the associated arthritis and spondylitis quite well.

Appendix 1
Ankylosing spondylitis organizations

International

The Ankylosing Spondylitis International Federation (ASIF) is a worldwide organization of national self-help societies for people suffering from AS or related diseases. It was established in 1988 to increase public awareness and knowledge of these diseases around the world and maintains a home page on the Internet: *www.asif.rheumanet.org*

The aims of ASIF are:

- exchange of information and experiences among the member societies
- cooperation in international research projects
- exchange of articles for publication in the journals of the member societies
- support of the development of newly formed societies
- establishment of contacts with AS patients in countries where an AS society does not yet exist.

National and local

There are many such support groups and organizations in various countries. Their aims are to:

- contribute to the physical and mental health of patients with AS or related diseases
- organize supervised exercise and recreational therapy groups throughout each country
- arrange the exchange of experiences among the patients
- oppose the social isolation of the patients
- advise patients regarding social, medical and work-related problems associated with their disease
- cooperate with doctors and allied health professionals
- represent the interests of the patients in the society, including the legislature (law) and the health services
- promote and encourage scientific research of the diseases
- increase public awareness and disseminate knowledge of the diseases in their respective regions or countries.

These societies are listed below. However, addresses (including homepage and e-mail addresses) and telephone and fax numbers do change from time to time. An up-to-date list is maintained by ASIF on their Internet home page, *www.asif.rheumanet.org*

Useful information can also be obtained through Internet home pages, such as *www.spondylitis.org* (based in the USA) and *www.nass.co.uk* (based in the UK). These and many of the other support groups listed below enlist enthusiastic patient co-operation, and provide useful information, booklets and pamphlets about AS and related spondylo-arthropathies for the people with AS and their families. Many of them can also provide advice about useful items such as wide-view mirrors for cars, working environment, insurance needs, jobs, exercises, and so on.

Australia

Ankylosing Spondylitis Group of New South Wales
PO Box 95, Artarmon, New South Wales 2064
Tel. (0061) 2 9412 2505
Email: asgroupnsw@ozemail.com.au

Ankylosing Spondylitis Group of Queensland
PO Box 7366, East Brisbane, Queensland 4169
Tel. (0061) 7 3391 4689
Email: asgroupld@arthritis.org.au
Internet homepage: *www.arthritis.org.au/asgroup*

Ankylosing Spondylitis Group of Western Australia
35 Wesley Street, Balcatta, Western Australia 6021
Tel. (0061) 9 344 5857

Austria

Österreichische Vereinigung Morbus Bechterew (ÖVMB)
Obere Augartenstr. 26–28, A-1020 Wien
Tel. (Mi 15–17h) and Fax: (0043) 1 33 22 810
Email: gesch@bechterew.at
Internet homepage: *www.bechterew.at*

Belgium (Flanders)

Vlaamse Vereniging voor Bechterew-patiënten (VVB)
c/o Leopold Bogaert, Pinksterbloemhof 16, 8300-Knokke-Heist
Tel. (0032) 50 51 28 30
Email: coby@village.uunet.be
Internet homepage: *www.vvb.rheumanet.org*

Canada

Ankylosing Spondylitis Association of British Columbia (ASABC)
2532 Western Avenue, North Vancouver, BC, Canada V7N 3 L1
Email: painsolv@smartt.com

Manitoba Ankylosing Spondylitis Association
c/o Lorne Ferley, 19 Carolyn Bay, Winnipeg, Manitoba, Canada R2J 2Z3,
Tel. (001-204) 256–53 20, Fax (001-204) 231 19 12

Ontario Spondylitis Association (OSA)
393 University Avenue, Suite 1700, Toronto, Ontario, Canada M5G 1E6

Tel. (001-416) 979-7228, Fax (001-416) 979-8366
Email (Arthritis Society): jwright@on.arthritis.ca
Internet homepage of Arthritis Society: *www.arthritis.ca*

Croatia

Hrvatsko društvo za ankilozantni spondilitis (a section of Croatian League against Rheumatism)
Prof. Ivo Jajic, Vinogradska c. 29, HR-10000 Zagreb
Tel. (00385-1) 37 87 248, Fax (00385-1) 37 69 067

Czech Republic

Klub bechtěreviků
c/o Revmatologicky ústav, Na Slupi 4, 128 50 Praha 2
Tel./Fax (00420-2) 69 13 870
Internet homepage: *www.radio.cz/rhs/klubb*

Denmark

Landsforeningen af Morbus Bechterew Patienter
v/ Advokat Per Lignell, Rosenvænget 58, DK-8362 Hørning
Tel. (0045) 86 92 33 00, Fax (0045) 86 92 30 65,
Email: plignell@post3.tele.dk

Germany

Deutsche Vereinigung Morbus Bechterew (DVMB)
Metzgergasse 16, D-97421 Schweinfurt
Tel. (09721) 22033, Fax (09721) 22955
Email: dvmb@talknet.de,
Internet homepage: *www.dvmb.rheumanet.org*

Great Britain (UK)

National Ankylosing Spondylitis Society (NASS)
PO Box 179, Mayfield, East Sussex TN20 6ZL
Tel. (0044-1435) 873527, Fax (0044-1435) 873027
Email: nass@nass.co.uk,
Internet homepage: *www.nass.co.uk*

Hungary

Mozgáskorlátozottak Egyesületeinek Országos Szövetsége, Bechterew section
c/o Dr.-Ing. Majtényi Sándor, Zrinyi utca 109/B, H-1196 Budapest
Tel. + Fax (0036-1) 280 38 30

Ireland

Ankylosing Spondylitis Association of Ireland (ASAI)
c/o Mr. Seoirse Smith, 6 Falcarragh Road, Gaeltacht Park, Whitehall,
Dublin 9
Tel. (+353-1) 83 76 614
Email: seopax@oceanfree.net

Italy

Associazione Italiana Spondiloartrite Anchilosante (A.I.Sp.A)
c/o Favio Fornasari, Via Elisabetta Sirani, 3/2, I-40129 Bologna
Tel./Fax (0039-51) 37 23 23

Japan

Japan Ankylosing Spondylitis Club
c/o Dr. Inoue Hisashi, 1-11-5, Shinkawa Mitaka-shi, Tokyo 181-0004
Tel. (0081-422) 45-79 85, Fax (0081-422) 49-68 17

Netherlands

*Nederlandse bond van verenigingen van patiënten met reumatische
aandoeningen, Commissie Morbus Bechterew*
Postbus 1370, 3800 BJ Amersfoort
Tel. (0031-33) 61 63 64, Fax (0031-33) 65 12 00

Norway

Norsk Revmatikerforbund (NRF)/Bekhterev
Postboks 2653 Solli, N-0203 Oslo
Tel. (0047) 22 55 72 16, Fax (0047) 22 43 12 51
Email: nrf.adm@rheuma.no,
Internet homepage: *www.rheuma.no*

Portugal

Associação Nacional da Espondilite Anquilosante (ANEA)
Rua Fernando Ribeiro, n: 57, P-2645-094 Alcabideche
Tel. (00351-21) 46 02 511, Fax (00351-21) 46 02 509
Email: anea@mail.telepac.pt
Internet homepage: *www.terravista.pt/mussulo/2553*

Slovenia

Društvo za ankilozirajoči spondilitis Slovenije (DASS)
c/o Marjan Hudomalj, Parmova 53, SI-1000 Ljubljana
Tel. (00386-61) 159 30 21, Fax (00386-61) 159 35 02
Email: dbiass@guest.arnes.si
Internet homepage: *www.drustvo-as.si*

Spain

Coordinadora Nacional de Espondilitis anquilosante
c/o Liga Reumatológica Española (LIRE), C/ Cid 4-1º, Apartado 112,
E-28001 Madrid
Tel. (0034-1) 914358132 und (0034-1) 902113188
Email: fepamic@mx2.redestb.es
Asociación Cordobesa de Enfermos Afectados de Espondilitis (ACEADE)
Apartado de Correos 762, E-14080 Córdoba

Sweden

Bechterewreumatikernas Intresseorganisation (BERI)
Seglaregatan 29 / Box 12031, S-402 41 Göteborg
Tel. (Mo-Fr 10-15) (0046-31)147 147, Fax (0046-31) 122 305

Switzerland

Schweizerische Vereinigung Morbus Bechterew (SVMB)
Röntgenstr. 22, CH-8005 Zürich
Tel. (0041-1) 272 78 66, Fax (0041-1) 272 78 75
Email: mail@bechterew.ch
Internet homepage: *www.bechterew.ch*

Singapore

Singapore Ankylosing Spondylitis Club (SASC)
c/o National Arthritis Foundation, 336 Smith Street, #06-302 New
Bridge Centre, Singapur 050336
Tel. (0065) 227-97 26, Fax (0065) 227-02 57
Internet homepage: *www.ttsh.gov.sg/medical/as/*

Taiwan

Ankylosing Spondylitis Caring Society of R.O C.
Dr Hwa-Chang Liu, Department of Orthopaedic Surgery, National
Taiwan University Hospital, 7 Chung-Shan South Road, Taipei
Tel. (00886-2) 397 08 00 Ext. 5688, Fax (00886-2) 395 69 88
Email: wei3228@ms3.hinet.net
Internet homepages: *www.health.nsysu.edu.tw/wei/as* and
www.ascare.org.tw

Ukraine

Society of Patients with Ankylosing Spondylitis (Bechterew's disease),
Bechterew group in Solotonosha
c/o Osirskij Viktor Dmitrijewich), Boulevard Gagarina 13/8,
Solotonosha, Ukraine 258100
Tel. (+380-475) 83 34, Fax (+380-475) 2172

USA

Spondylitis Association of America (SAA)
PO Box 5872, Sherman Oaks, CA 91413
Tel. (001-818) 981-1616, Fax (001-818) 981-9826
Email: info@spondylitis.org
Internet homepage: *www.spondylitis.org*

Research organizations

Anyone interested in research studies in North America can contact
the following organizations:

Spondylitis Association of America (SAA)
PO Box 5872, Sherman Oaks, CA 91413
Tel. (001-818) 981-1616, Fax (001-818) 981-9826
Email: info@spondylitis.org,
Internet homepage: *www.spondylitis.org*

North American Spondylitis Consortium (NASC)
Internet homepage: *www.asresearch.org*

In Europe research studies into AS have also been under way for some years. Interested families there can contact the following organizations: Wellcome Trust Centre for Human Genetics, Oxford, England Consortium Européen pour les études génétiques et immunogénétiques de la Spondalarthrite Ankylosante et des autres Spondylarthropathies with research partners in Belgium, Finland, France, Germany, Great Britain, Italy, Portugal, and Sweden.

Internet-based rheumatology education

www.rheuma21st.com
http://rheuma.bham.ac.uk
www.jointandbone.org
www.nlm.nih.gov/medlineplus

Appendix 2
Glossary

Achilles tendinitis inflammation of the Achilles tendon, causing swelling and tenderness at the lower end of the calf where it inserts into the heel bone

acupuncture an ancient medical procedure that originated in China more than 2000 years ago. It is based on the theoretical concept of balanced Qi (pronounced 'chee') or vital energy that flows throughout the body via certain pathways that are accessed by puncturing the skin with hair-thin needles at particular locations called **acupuncture points**. Stimulation of acupuncture points is believed to stimulate the brain and spinal cord to release chemicals that change the experience of pain or cause biochemical changes that may stimulate healing and promote general well-being. See also **alternative and complementary remedies; traditional Chinese medicine**

allele alternate forms of a gene at a distinct location (locus) on a chromosome

alternative and complementary remedies these include holistic medicine, folk remedies, and alternative therapies (herbal medications or extracts, homeopathy, Ayurvedics, and traditional Chinese medicine (TCM). These complementary and alternative treatments are mostly based on anecdotal evidence, primarily from individuals who report their own successful use of the treatment. One needs to apply scientific methods to establish the validity of the anecdotal evidence

amino acids   small organic molecules which are the building blocks of peptides and proteins

amyloid   a proteinaceous fibrillar material deposited in various tissues and organs, sometimes secondary to a chronic inflammatory disease

analgesia   pain relief, e.g. by such drugs as paracetamol, **NSAIDs** or narcotics. These pain-relieving drugs are called **analgesics** (see NSADs)

ankylosing hyperostosis   also called **Forestier's disease** or **diffuse idiopathic skeletal hyperostosis** (DISH). It causes excessive new bone formation along the spine and other sites (at entheses), can result in stiff spine that may be confused with AS

ankylosing spondylitis (AS)   an inflammatory arthritic disorder, primarily of the axial skeleton (sacroiliac joints and spine), but can affect hip and shoulder joints and infrequently the peripheral joints. It causes chronic back pain and leads to stiffness of the spine. Most of the affected individuals have the HLA-B27 gene

ankylosis   fusion, which may be fibrous, or bony (as in AS)

annulus fibrosus   the tough outer fibrous layer of the intervertebral disc

antibodies   proteins produced by white blood cells (plasma cells and B lymphocytes) that confer immunity

antigen   a substance that causes the body's immune system to produce antibodies that try to eliminate it because the body sees the antigen as foreign or harmful substance (e.g. from invading viruses or bacteria)

antigen-presenting cell   a cell that ingests and processes foreign substance (e.g. from invading viruses or bacteria) and displays the resulting antigen fragments (small peptides) on its surface to activate those T cells that respond specifically to that antigen

aortitis inflammation of the aorta, which is the main artery that carries the blood from the heart to ultimately supply the needs of the body

arachnoiditis fibrosis (scarring) of the membrane covering the spinal cord and spinal nerve roots as they pass through the spinal canal. This results in entrapment of these nerve roots that may cause chronic back and leg pain and neurological dysfunction. It can occur following spinal surgery, and has also been associated in the past with the use of an X-ray contrast medium. Very rarely it can occur in the lower end of the spinal canal in AS without any apparent reason, and is the cause of **cauda equina syndrome** in this disease

arthralgia pain in one or more joints without any outward evidence of a joint abnormality

arthritis literally means inflammation of the joint, and is used to refer to more than 100 joint diseases, some of which may also affect other regions of the body. The plural is **arthritides**

arthritis mutilans an extremely destructive form of arthritis; the term is usually applied to a very severe form of psoriatic arthritis

arthrocentesis taking a sample of joint fluid out for testing, obtained by a needle puncture of the joint. Sometimes all of the joint fluid may be aspirated as a part of treatment

arthrodesis a surgically induced or spontaneous fusion of a joint

arthroplasty surgical procedure to alter a joint, e.g. its excision and replacement by an artificial joint

arthroscopy inspection of the inside of a joint, e.g. for obtaining a biopsy, usually through a fiber optic instrument called **arthroscope**

autoimmune disease a disease in which the immune system attacks and destroys the body's own tissues that it mistakenly believes to be foreign

axial arthritis   arthritis in the spine and/or neighboring joints, especially the sacroiliac joints, as in AS, in contrast to arthritis of peripheral (limb) joints

Ayurveda   the traditional Indian medical system, which claims that health is based on a harmonious relationship between three humors called 'doshas', and disharmony results in disease

B cells (B lymphocytes)   antibody-producing white blood cells, which mature in the bone marrow. The letter B originally came from bursa of Fabricius where B lymphocytes originate in chickens, but has subsequently been extended to imply the bone marrow

bamboo spine   X-ray appearance of spine in advanced AS because of spinal fusion producing a bamboo-like appearance

biologic response modifiers   drugs which are also called **biologicals** for short, and include anti-TNF drugs infliximab (Remicade) and etanercept (Enbrel)

biopsy   removal of a small tissue specimen for examination

bisphosphonates   drugs used to treat osteoporosis because they inhibit bone resorption

bowel   a word commonly used for the small and large intestines (see **gut; large intestine; small intestine**)

brand name   the brand name (trademark) of a drug is coined by the manufacturer in agreement with the regulating agencies, unlike the **generic name** which indicates its active ingredients. For example, celecoxib is the generic name for the drug whose brand name is Celebrex. The brand name starts with a capital letter but the generic name does not. Several brand name drugs can have the same generic name if they contain the same active ingredient. Thus, Motrin and Aleve are both brand names for the generic drug ibuprofen

bursa   a fluid-filled sac found between tissue planes over bony places subject to shearing forces, as over the elbow and knee. It is lined by synovium that secretes the lubricating fluid

bursitis   an inflammation of a bursa

calcification   deposition of chalky (calcific) material in tissue, leading to bone formation

Campylobacter   a type of bacteria. Enteric infections with these bacteria can trigger reactive arthritis in susceptible individuals

capsule   a thick membrane joining together ends of two adjacent bones to form a joint. Its inside is lined with synovium that forms the joint fluid

cartilage   a tissue that covers the ends of bones to form a smooth shock-absorbing surface for joints, and results in very low friction movement. Cartilage also occurs at other sites, such as the nose and the ears

cauda equina syndrome   some people with advanced AS on rare occasions may get this neurological condition resulting from gradual scarring at the lower end of the spine that entraps the lower spinal nerves. The name cauda equina means horsetail, so named because the lowermost spinal nerves slope downward as a bunch before they exit the vertebral column.

CD4+ (CD8+) T lymphocytes   these T cells carry a marker on the surface known as a cluster of differentiation (CD) marker which can be either CD4 or CD8. The CD4+ T cells, also known as **helper T cells**, help orchestrate the antibody responses, and the CD8+ T cells—also called **cytotoxic** (destructive to cells) or **suppressor T cells**—are involved in cell-mediated immunity that targets infected cells

celiac disease   inability to digest and absorb a protein found in wheat, resulting in poor absorption of nutrients from the foods because of damage to the lining of the small intestine; also called gluten intolerance or non-tropical sprue

cervicitis   inflammation of the cervix, the part of the uterus that protrudes into the vagina

chromosome a thread-like structure within the nucleus of a cell that contains the genes. There are 46 chromosomes in the nucleus of a human cell; 22 of them are in pairs that are given the numbers 1–22, and the remaining two are the X or Y chromosomes (sex chromosomes) that determine a person's sex—males have one X and one Y chromosomes, and females have two X chromosomes

Chlamydia trachomatis a bacterium that has a predilection to infect the genitourinary tract. Such an infection is the more commonly recognized initiator of reactive arthritis in the US

Clostridium difficile bacteria that are normally present in the large intestine, can cause a serious illness called pseudo-membranous colitis in people taking antibiotics, and can sometimes trigger reactive arthritis

collagen and connective tissue a set of fibrous proteins and supporting framework that form the main building blocks of the body, including the internal organs, ligaments, tendon, cartilage, bone, and skin

conjunctivitis commonly known as **pink eye**; it is an inflammation of the delicate outer membrane that lines the inside of the eyelids and the white of the eye

contracture arthritis or prolonged immobility can result in the involved joint becoming less freely moveable. Associated with shortening and wasting of muscles

control group in clinical studies the control group, which is given either the standard treatment for a medical condition under study or an inactive substance (called a **placebo**), is compared with a group given an experimental treatment to find its efficacy for the disease under study

coping the psychological processes following any stressful situation

cortisone a natural hormone made by the adrenal gland. Sometimes wrongly used as a synonym for corticosteroids

corticosteroids   a group of related compounds which, like cortisone, reduce inflammation and irritation caused by many disease processes, including many forms of arthritis, and skin and bowel diseases

Crohn's disease   a chronic inflammatory bowel disease (also called ileitis or regional enteritis), that can affect the entire gastrointestinal tract, though it usually involves the lower small intestine, (the ileum) and the adjacent part of the colon

C-reactive protein (CRP)   its measurement in the blood can be used to detect or grade inflammation

cytokine   a soluble protein, produced by white blood cells, that acts as a messenger between cells, either stimulating or inhibiting the activity of various cells of the immune system. There is normally a very delicate balance among the various cytokines

cytoplasm   a liquid compartment in the cell, surrounding the central nucleus. The cytoplasm contains mitochondria and other structures or components responsible for normal protein formation, secretion and other cell functions

DEXA bone scan   a means of measuring the bone density to detect osteoporosis at a much earlier stage as compared to a standard X-ray. DEXA stands for dual-energy X-ray absorption i.e. X-ray absorption at two different quantum energies or wavelengths

disorder   a synonym for disease

disability   in the context of health experience, a disability is a restriction or lack (resulting from an impairment) of ability to perform an activity in the manner or within the range considered normal (see WHO, 1980)

distal   farther away from the trunk. For example, a hand is the distal end of an arm. The opposite is **proximal**

DNA   a double-stranded, helical molecule that carries genetic information, primarily present within the nucleus of each cell in plants and animals. It tells the cells exactly what to do and how to perform their functions

double-blinded   a doubled-blinded trial produces more objective and unbiased results because neither the research investigators nor the study participants know who is receiving the investigational drug and who is receiving the placebo

duodenum   the first part of the small intestine. An ulcer on its inner lining is called a **duodenal ulcer**

dowager's hump   hump in the upper back (thoracic kyphosis) in an elderly woman with osteoporosis

dysentery   an infectious disease of the intestine that causes bloody, mucus-filled diarrhea, which can be accompanied by abdominal pain or cramps, fever, and dehydration from excessive diarrhea. It is caused by enteric infections, usually with *Shigella*, and can sometimes trigger reactive arthritis

elimination diet   requirement that certain foods should not be eaten

enteritis   an inflammation (irritation) of the small intestine

enthesis   site of attachment of ligament or tendon to bone

enthesitis   inflammation of an enthesis

enthesopathy   an all-inclusive term that covers all abnormalities of an enthesis (e.g. enthesitis is an inflammatory type of enthesopathy)

enzyme   a protein that acts to promote or facilitate certain biochemical processes in the body; e.g. many enzymes produced in the gut assist in digestion of food

epicondylitis   enthesopathy at bony prominence (epicondyle) of the elbow; may occur on the medial (inner) side (golfer's elbow) or the lateral (outer) side (tennis elbow)

erythrocyte sedimentation rate (ESR)   a blood test commonly used to detect or grade inflammation

esophagus   the tube-like passage through which swallowed food travels from the mouth to the stomach

familial   a term used to indicate a disease or a trait (an inherited characteristic) which tends to affect more than one member in a family

fascia   tough membrane that encloses muscles and other organs

fasciitis   inflammation of the fascia.

fibromyalgia   a complex chronic painful condition, primarily occurring in women, characterized by widespread musculoskeletal pain, and fatigue, and accompanied by tender points at defined locations, often associated with a non-restorative sleep pattern

fibrositis   a term used interchangeably with **fibromyalgia**

folic acid and **folinic acid**   members of the vitamin B complex

food poisoning   an acute food-borne gastrointestinal infection caused by food contaminated by harmful bacteria that results in symptoms such as diarrhea, abdominal discomfort or cramps, and fever

Forestier's disease   see **ankylosing hyperostosis**

gastric ulcer   an ulcer on the inner lining of the stomach

gastrointestinal tract   alimentary tract, including esophagus, stomach, duodenum, ileum, large bowel, and rectum

gene   part of the **DNA** molecule responsible for making proteins. It is the basic unit of heredity; all information in the genes (genetic information) is passed from parent to child

generic name   see **brand name**

genetic counseling   informing people about genetic facts that may guide them in making a decision based on a knowledge of disease risk. The word **genetic** refers to any characteristic that is inherited

genetic marker   a gene that is used to identify an individual disease or trait, or trace its inheritance within a family

genitourinary tract   the genitalia, the bladder, and the urethral tube through which the bladder empties

gut   a word in common use to describe the large and small intestine (see **bowel, large intestine; small intestine**)

handicap   in the context of health experience, a handicap is a disadvantage for a given individual, resulting from an impairment or a disability, that limits or prevents the fulfillment of a role that is normal (depending on age, sex, and social and cultural factors) for that individual (see WHO, 1980)

H2-blockers   medicines such as cimetidine (Tagamet), ranitidine (Zantac), or famotidine (Pepcid), used to treat acid indigestion, heartburn, and ulcer pain. They are so called because they act by blocking histamine-2 signals to reduce the amount of acid produced by the stomach

heartburn   symptoms caused by stomach acid flowing back into the **esophagus**

Helicobacter pylori   a corkscrew-shaped bacterium found in the stomach that can predispose to stomach and duodenal ulcers. Previously called *Campylobacter pylori*

heterozygote and **homoozygote**   an individual inherits a set of two **alleles** for each HLA locus from his or her parents. For instance, an individual may inherit HLA-B27 from one parent and HLA-B8 from the other. Most individuals do not inherit the same gene (belonging to a locus) from both parents, and are said to be **heterozygotes**. Someone who inherits the same gene, e.g. HLA-B27, from both parents is **homozygous** for HLA-B27

HLA   human leucocyte antigens. These are cell surface proteins, detected by blood testing, that vary from person to person. They are also called tissue antigens or histocompatibility antigens because ideally organ donors and recipients must have compatible HLA;

otherwise the transplanted organ is recognized as non-self ('foreign') and is rejected. HLA are related to the workings of the immune system; they present self- and foreign-derived (e.g. viral) peptides (a few amino acids linked together) to T lymphocytes and other cells of the immune system that help the body fight illness. They are of two broad types, called class I and class II HLA. Their genes are located on chromosome 6; the loci are given the letters A, B, C, D, and so on

HLA-B27 an HLA class I molecule that has been assigned the number 27; its gene is present at the B locus. There are quite a few HLA antigens that confer susceptibility to certain diseases: HLA-B27 to AS, and HLA-DR4 to rheumatoid arthritis, for example

hydrotherapy physiotherapy in a pool (usually heated)

idiopathic of unknown cause or explanation

ileum the major part of the small intestine (see small intestine)

ilium (or iliac bone) major bony component of the pelvis. There is one on each side, joined to the sacrum via the right and left sacroiliac joints

impairment in the context of health experience, an impairment is any loss or abnormality of psychological, physiological or anatomical structure or function (WHO, 1980)

incidence the rate of occurrence of some event, such as the number of individuals who get a disease divided by a total given population, per unit of time (usually per year). In contrast to **prevalence**, incidence describes the number of new cases of a disease among a certain group of people for a certain period of time, i.e. how often a new case is diagnosed

inflammation a typical reaction of tissues to injury or disease, usually marked by four signs: pain, swelling, redness, and heat. It may be acute (as in a burn or in gouty arthritis) or chronic (as in rheumatoid arthritis or chronic infections such as tuberculosis)

inflammatory bowel disease   a chronic (long-lasting) inflammatory disease of the gut, e.g. ulcerative colitis or Crohn's disease

internist   a doctor specializing in internal medicine (not requiring surgery).

intestine   also called **bowel** or **gut** (see **large intestine; small intestine**)

intestinal flora   bacteria and other organisms that normally grow in the intestine

intestinal mucosa   surface lining of the intestines where the absorption of nutrients takes place.

intra-articular   into or within a joint, e.g. intra-articular injection

joint   the place where two bones meet. Most joints are composed of cartilage, joint space, fibrous capsule, joint lining (synovium) and ligaments

juvenile chronic arthritis   arthritis in children 16 years of age or less, that has been present for at least 3 months, and for which no other cause is obvious. It is now preferably called **juvenile idiopathic arthritis**

keratoderma blennorrhagica   rash on palms of the hands and soles of the feet which may occur in reactive arthritis (Reiter's syndrome); it resembles a form of psoriasis

kyphosis   forward stooping (bowing) of the spine ('humpback' deformity)

large intestine   part of the intestine that changes stool from a liquid to a solid form by absorbing water. Often simply called the **colon**, but in fact includes the appendix, cecum, colon, and rectum; has a total length of about 5 feet (1.5 m).

leukocyte   white blood cell, part of the immune system

ligament   stretchy tough band of cord-like tissue that connects bones together, and confers stability by restraining excessive joint movement

limb girdle joints   hip and shoulder joints

locus   precise location of a gene on a chromosome

lymphocyte   a type of white blood cell present in the blood, lymph and lymphoid tissues; primarily responsible for immune responses (see also **B lymphocytes; CD4+ (CD8+) T lymphocytes; T lymphocytes**)

macrophage   a relatively large immune system cell that devours invading bacteria and other intruders, and stimulates other immune cells by presenting them with small pieces of the invaders. Can sometimes harbor large quantities of invading viruses like HIV without being killed, and thus act as a reservoir of such viruses

magnetic resonance imaging (MRI)   a method of taking pictures of the soft tissues in the body that are clearer than those obtained by X-rays, and without radiation

medial   on the inside (as opposed to **lateral**); not to be confused with the **median** nerve which is compressed in carpal tunnel syndrome

methotrexate   a drug which is used in low doses for the treatment of inflammatory disorders, including various types of inflammatory arthritis, and in very high doses to treat certain cancers. It is sometimes abbreviated to MTX (See also **slow-acting anti-rheumatic drugs**)

monoclonal antibodies   artificially produced antibodies used in research and also for treatment of some diseases. They are produced in a cell culture (clone) by multiplying one single mother cell thus having exactly the same properties (very pure antibody)

MRI   See **magnetic resonance imaging**

nucleus   the central controlling structure within a living cell that contains the genetic codes (in chromosomes) for maintaining life systems of the cell and for issuing commands for cell growth and reproduction

nausea   the feeling of wanting to throw up (vomit)

neurohormones   biochemical substances made by tissue in the body's nervous system that can change the function or structure, or direct the activity of tissues or organs; e.g. neurotransmitters

neurological   relating to the body's nervous system, which oversees and controls all body functions

neurotransmitters   biochemical substances that stimulate or inhibit nerve impulses in the brain that relay information about external stimuli and sensations, such as pain

NK (natural killer) cells   non-specific lymphocytes like killer T cells that attack and kill cancer and infected cells. They are natural killers because they do not need to recognize a specific antigen in order to attack and kill

NSAID (non-steroidal anti-inflammatory drug)   non-cortisone, non-addictive (non-narcotic) drug that reduces pain and inflammation and is therefore used in the treatment of pain and arthritis

oligoarthritis   inflammation of up to four joints; if more joints are involved, then the disease is called **polyarthritis**

onycholysis   nail abnormality and discoloration seen in psoriasis and reactive arthritis; may be accompanied by pitting of the nail in psoriasis.

Osgood–Schlatter's disease   a childhood condition of the site of attachment of the patellar (kneecap) tendon into the tibial tubercle, a bony prominence an inch or so below the kneecap. Results in localized pain and tenderness that can sometimes be confused with enthesitis at this site seen in some children with juvenile AS and related diseases

osteitis condensans ilii   increased bone density (sclerosis) at the sacral side of the sacroiliac joint that is of unknown cause and is usually without symptoms. Its X-ray appearance can be confused with sacroiliitis

osteoarthritis (osteoarthrosis)   degenerative disorder of joints, most often from disease in the spine and in the weight bearing joints (knees and hips). Normally seen with aging, but can occur prematurely due to various reasons, for instance after an injury to a joint. Also known as **degenerative joint disease**, it can cause joint pain, loss of function, reduced joint motion, and deformity

osteomalacia   bone-thinning disorder resulting from deficiency of vitamin D. Can be mistaken for osteoporosis, and can also be confused with spondylitis. The childhood form of osteomalacia is called **rickets**

osteophyte   bony outgrowth (seen on X-ray) at joint margin of an osteoarthritic joint, or in degenerative disc disease

osteoporosis   a disease characterized by reduction in mineral content usually seen with aging, but also in connection with certain conditions such as paralysis, or due to prolonged use of certain drugs, such as corticosteroids

Paget's disease   a disease characterized by accelerated bone turnover, resulting in the involved bone becoming enlarged but weak and fragile. The bone also feels warmer to touch due to increased blood supply. Also called **osteitis deformans**

pathogenesis   process of development of a disease

pauciarthritis   same as **oligoarthritis**

pelvis   the bony structures in the lowest part of the trunk. The term **pelvic** is used for anything that belongs or refers to the pelvis

peptic ulcer   a sore in the lining of the stomach (**gastric ulcer**) or duodenum (**duodenal ulcer**). The word peptic refers to the stomach and the duodenum, where pepsin is present, an enzyme that breaks down proteins. An ulcer can sometimes occur in the lower part of the esophagus in association with heartburn.

peptide   a few amino acids linked together. Proteins are made of multiple peptides linked together

placebo   originally a Latin word meaning 'I will please'. Now used for inactive substance (sham) given to participants of a research study in order to test the efficacy of another substance or treatment. In short-term clinical trials, many of the most valued drugs in clinical use are only about 25% more effective than placebo. Scientists often have to compare the effects of active and inactive substances to learn more about how the active substance affects participants; in such studies both doctor and patient are unaware of who is receiving the active or inactive substance. Such studies are known as **double blind placebo controlled** studies

polyarthralgia   pains in many joints; conventionally refers to more than four joints, without signs of inflammation in the symptomatic joints

polyarthritis   inflammation in many joints; conventionally in more than four joints

preclinical diagnosis   diagnosis of a genetic disease before there are any symptoms or signs

prevalence   the observed number of people in a given population affected with a particular disease or condition at a given time, usually stated as the number of cases observed per 100 000 individuals, or listed as a percentage. In contrast with **incidence**, prevalence can be thought of as a snapshot of all existing cases at a specified time

prognosis   the probable end result or outcome of a disease

protein   a large molecule composed of amino acids. Essential components of the body tissue (see also **peptide**)

proton pump inhibitors   a group of drugs used to treat heartburn and peptic ulcer disease. These include omprezole (Prilosec), esomeprazole (Nexium) and pansoprazole (Prevacid)

prospective, randomized, double blind study   clinical trial or study in which the method of data analysis is specified in a protocol before the study is begun (prospective). Patients are randomly assigned to receive either the study drug or an alternative treatment, and neither the patient nor the doctor conducting the study knows which treatment is being given to which patient (see also **placebo**)

proximal   the part of a limb that is closest to the trunk. For example, the shoulder joint forms the proximal end of the upper extremity (opposite of **distal**)

psoriasis   a common chronic skin disease, more common in whites (2% of the population) than in other racial groups, in which red flaky lesions occur—often on the elbows and knees, or in the scalp. May cause nail abnormalities

psoriatic arthritis   arthritis associated with psoriasis; occurs in more than 10% of people with psoriasis. May occur in several forms

Qi   Chinese term for vital energy or life force. Pronounced chee (see **acupuncture**)

radiography/radiograph/radiogram/radiologic   radiography (or roentgenography) is the method of taking a picture with the help of X-rays, and the terms radiograph or simply X-ray are sometimes used for the resulting picture. Radiogram is the correct name for an image taken by radiography

randomized, double-blind, placebo-controlled, multicenter trial   a clinical trial in which patients have been randomly assigned to receive either the study drug or the alternative treatment under study. Neither the patient nor the doctor conducting the study knows which treatment is being given; the alternative to the study drug is a placebo; and the study is conducted at several centers

range of motion   the extent to which a joint is able to go through all of its normal movements. Range-of-motion exercises help increase or maintain flexibility and movement in muscles, tendons, ligaments, and joints

reactive arthritis   arthritis resulting from infection elsewhere in the body; i.e. there is no infection in the joint. The commonest type is HLA B27-related and may follow certain types of bowel or genitourinary infection

Reiter's syndrome a form of HLA B27-related reactive arthritis with a classical triad of arthritis, conjunctivitis, and urethritis, with or without other features of spondyloarthropathies. The term **reactive arthritis** is now used more commonly to describe this condition

rheumatic fever a form of reactive arthritis triggered by streptococcal sore throat. Its features include very painful joint inflammation (arthritis). It is now uncommon in developed countries but still occurs commonly in other parts of the world. It can cause inflammation and scarring of heart valvos (rheumatic heart disease)

rheumatoid arthritis a chronic systemic disease that causes inflammatory changes in the synovium, or joint lining, that result in pain, stiffness, swelling, and ultimately loss of function and deformities of the affected joints due to destruction of the cartilage and adjacent bone. The disease can also affect other parts of the body. In the past it was also called **chronic polyarthritis**. It is more common in women than men, and at least 70% of patients show a positive blood test for **rheumatoid factor**

rheumatologist a doctor (board-certified internist or pediatrician) who has had specialized training in diagnosing and treating disorders that affect the joints, muscles, tendons, ligaments, connective tissue, and bones

roentgenography see **radiography**

sacroiliac joints two joints, one on either side, in the lower back, between the two pelvic bones called sacrum and ilium (see Figure 4)

sacroiliitis inflammation of the sacroiliac joint; bilateral sacroiliitis is a hallmark of AS

sacrum major bony component of the pelvis, shaped like a wedge on which the spine rests. It forms a joint

with ilium, one on each side, via the right and left
sacroiliac joints

Salmonella a group of bacteria comprising many different types that may cause intestinal infection and
diarrhea called **salmonellosis**, which includes typhoid
fever. Enteric infections with *Salmonella*, *Shigella*,
Yersinia, or *Campylobacter* are the most common triggers for reactive arthritis, especially in some developing
parts of the world

SAPHO syndrome so named because of its salient features: **s**ynovitis, **a**cne, **p**almoplantar pustulosis, **h**yperostosis, aseptic **o**steomyelitis. This rare disease causes
aseptic (no evidence of infection) bone necrosis at
multiple sites that can include the sacroiliac joints or
the spine. It is known by many different names, but
SAPHO syndrome is the most common

sausage digit finger or toe that is diffusely swollen as a
result of tenosynovitis; usually seen in psoriatic and
reactive arthritis. It is also called dactylitis

Scheuermann's disease a non-inflammatory spinal
disease that occurs in adolescence and affects the
thoracic spine, especially the discs. Often painless, but
can result in a stooped back

Schober's test to detect the ability to bend forward
(flexibility) of the lumbar spine (see Figure 5g and
accompanying caption)

scoliosis a non-inflammatory rotational deformity of
the spine; results in a lateral curvature

selective estrogen receptor modulators (SERM) a
class of drugs used in the treatment of osteoporosis;
they mimic the effect of estrogen but in a tissue-
selective manner

septic arthritis bacterial infection of one or more
joints; requires urgent diagnosis and treatment

seronegative arthritis an arthritis that is not associated with the presence of an autoantibody called
rheumatoid factor in the blood. Most people with AS

and related spondyloarthopathies lack this auto-antibody, and therefore these diseases are examples of seronegative arthritis. On the other hand, only about 25% of people with rheumatoid arthritis are sero-negative

Shigella   a group of bacteria that can cause an illness called **shigellosis**, with high fever and acute diarrhea, sometimes mixed with blood (dysentery). Enteric infections with *Shigella* can trigger reactive arthritis

sibling   brother or sister

skeletal muscles   muscles that move the bony skeleton, i.e. provide movement at the joints

slit lamp   an instrument used by eye specialists (opthal-mologists) to look for inflammation or other diseases inside the eye

slow-acting and **symptom-modifying anti-rheumatic drugs (SAARDS** and **SMARDs)**   drugs such as sul-fasalazine and methotrexate, which may be useful in spondyloarthropathies that are resistant to conven-tional therapy. Any benefit from these drugs takes some time to manifest itself, hence the name. Unlike **NSAIDs**, these drugs are not pain relievers, but they will help relieve pain if they can first heal or control the underlying inflammation

small intestine   the tubular organ, about 20 feet (6 m) long, where most digestion occurs. It is made up of three parts: the **duodenum** (which is attached to the stomach), **jejunum**, and **ileum** (which ends in the **large intestine**)

spondylitis   literally means inflammation of the spine, and is best exemplified by ankylosing spondylitis (AS)

spondyloarthritis and **spondyloarthopathy**   AS and related diseases are grouped under this term. These diseases show clinical similarities to some extent, and occur much more often in people who carry the HLA-B27 gene

spondylolisthesis   a loss of spinal column alignment that results from one vertebra slipping forward on top of another

spondylosis   non-inflammatory degenerative (wear and tear) disease of the spinal column as we get older, such as degenerative disc disease

steroids   see **corticosteroids**

stomach ulcer   an open sore in the lining of the stomach. also called **gastric ulcer**

sulfasalazine   see **slow-acting anti-rheumatic drugs**

syndesmophytes   ligamentous bone deposits (ossification) producing fine bony bridging between adjacent vertebral bodies at the margin of the vertebrae, characteristic of AS. They are vertically orientated, unlike osteophytes (seen in degenerative disc disease), which grow horizontally

syndrome   a complex of signs and symptoms that when occurring together suggest a particular disease

synovium   a thin membrane (normally one or two cell layers thick) lining the inside of the joint capsule. It produces **synovial fluid** for lubrication and nourishment of the joint cartilage

synovitis   inflammation of the joints resulting from inflamed synovium; this results in joint inflammation (arthritis)

T cell (or T lymphocyte)   T stands for the thymus, where T lymphocytes mature. T cells are white blood cells that play a critical role in immune response, but, unlike B lymphocytes, do not produce antibodies (immunoglobulins). There are two main subtypes: the **CD4+ helper T cells** and the **CD8+ cytotoxic or suppressor T cells**

Tai Chi   a traditional Chinese mind–body relaxation exercise consisting of 108 intricate exercise sequences performed in a slow relaxed manner over a 30 minute period

temporo-mandibular joint (TMJ)   the jaw joint

tendon   a tough cord or band of fibrous tissue by which muscles are attached to bone

tendinitis (tendonitis)   inflammation of a tendon

TENS (transcutaneous electrical nerve stimulation)   a type of therapy used to relieve pain that involves passing electricity to nerve cells through electrodes placed on the skin

TNF (tumor necrosis factor alpha)   a **cytokine** (messenger protein) that plays a key role in the body's immune response by promoting inflammation, controlling the production of other pro-inflammatory molecules, and also helping the cells heal or repair themselves. It attaches to a cell surface protein called TNF receptor to exert its effect on the cell.

traditional Chinese medicine (TCM)   An ancient Chinese system of medicine, that includes meditation, herbal and nutritional therapy, restorative physical exercises and massage, and acupuncture. (See also **acupuncture; alternative healthcare and complementary remedies**)

urethritis   an inflammatory condition of the urethra (the tube through which the urine travels from the bladder to the outside during urination)

ulcer   a sore on the skin surface or on the inside lining of a body part, such as the mouth or stomach

ulcerative colitis   an inflammatory disease of the inner lining of the gut that usually involves the colon or rectum. (See also **inflammatory bowel disease**)

Yersinia   a group of bacteria comprising many different types that may cause intestinal infection and diarrhea. Enteric infections with *Yersinia*, *Salmonella*, *Shigella*, or *Campylobacter* are the most common triggers for reactive arthritis

References and further reading

Journal articles

Bakker C, Hidding A, van der Linden S, Doorslaer E van (1994) Cost effectiveness of group physical therapy compared to individualized therapy for ankylosing spondylitis. A randomized controlled trial. *Journal of Rheumatology* **21**: 264–268.

Ball J (1971) Enthesopathy of rheumatoid and ankylosing spondylitis. *Annals of Rheumatic Diseases* **30**: 213–223.

Banares A, Hernandez-Garcia C, Fernandez-Gutierrez B, Jover JA (1998) Eye involvement in the spondyloarthropathies. *Rheumatic Disease Clinics of North America* **24**: 771–784.

Barlow J, Cullen L (1996) Parenting and ankylosing spondylitis. Disability. *Pregnancy Parenthood International* **15**: 4–5.

Benedek TG, Rodnan GP (1982) A brief history of the rheumatic diseases. *Bulletin on the Rheumatic Diseases* **32**: 59–68.

Boyer GS, Templin DW, Bowler A and colleagues (1997) A comparison of patients with spondyloarthropathy seen in specialty clinics with those identified in a communitywide epidemiologic study. Has the classic case misled us? *Archives of Internal Medicine* **157**: 2111–2117.

Braun J, Brandt J, Listing J and colleagues (2002). Treatment of active ankylosing spondylitis with infliximab: a randomized controlled multicenter trial. *Lancet* **359**: 1187–1193.

Braun J, Bollow M, Reminger G and colleagues (1998) Prevalence of spondyloarthropathies in HLA-B27 positive and negative blood donors. *Arthritis and Rheumatism* **41**: 58–67.

Braun J, Bollow M, Sieper J (1998) Radiologic diagnosis and pathology of the spondyloarthropathies. *Rheumatic Disease Clinics of North America* **24**: 697–735.

Braun J, Khan MA, Sieper J (2000) Entheses and enthesopathy: What is the target of the immune response. *Annals of Rheumatic Diseases* **59**: 985–994.

Brus H, van der Laar M, Taal E, et al. (1997) Compliance in rheumatoid arthritis and the role of formal education. *Seminars in Arthritis and Rheumatism* **26**: 702–710.

Bulstrode SJ, Barefoot J, Harrison RA, Clarke AK (1987) The role of passive stretching in the treatment of ankylosing spondylitis. *British Journal of Rheumatology* **26**: 40–42.

Calin A, Nakache J-P, Gueguen A, Zeidler H, Mielants H, Dougados M (1999) Defining disease activity in ankylosing spondylitis: is a combination of variables (Bath Ankylosing Spondylitis Disease Activity Index) an appropriate instrument? *Rheumatology* **38**: 878–882.

Callahan LF, Pincus T (1995) Mortality in the rheumatic diseases. *Arthritis Care Research* **2**: 1327–1332.

Court-Brown WM, Doll R (1965) Mortality from cancer and other causes after radiotherapy for ankylosing spondylitis. *British Medical Journal* **59**: 327–538.

Dalyan M, Guner A, Tuncer S, Bilgic A, Arasil T (1999) Disability in ankylosing spondylitis. *Disability Rehabilitation* 21: 74–79.

Dougados M, Revel M, Khan MA (1998) Spondylarthropathy treatment: Progress in medical treatment, physical therapy and rehabilitation. *Baillière's Clinical Rheumatology* 12: 717–736.

Dougados M, Linden S van der, Juhlin R *et al.* (1991) The European Spondyloarthropathy Study Group preliminary criteria for the classification of spondyloarthropathies. *Arthritis and Rheumatism* 34: 1218–1227.

Ebringer A, Wilson C (1996) The use of a low starch diet in the treatment of patients suffering from ankylosing spondylitis. *Clinical Rheumatology* 15 (Suppl 1): 62–66.

Feldtkeller E, Bruckel J, Khan MA (2000) Contributions of the ankylosing spondylitis patient advocacy groups to spondyloarthritis research. *Current Opinion in Rheumatology* 12: 239–247.

Feldtkeller E, Khan MA, van der Linden S, van der Heijde D, Braun J (submitted) Age at disease onset and diagnosis delay in HLA-B27 negative vs. positive ankylosing spondylitis. *Annals of Rheumatic Disease* (submitted)

Finkelstein JA, Chapman JR, Mirza S (1999) Occult vertebral fractures in ankylosing spondylitis. *Spinal Cord* 37: 444–447.

François RJ, Braun J, Khan MA (2001) Entheses and enthesitis: a histopathological review and relevance to spondyloarthritides. *Current Opinion in Rheumatology* 13: 255–264.

Franke A and colleagues (2000) Long-term efficacy of radon spa therapy in rheumatoid arthritis—a randomized, sham-controlled study and follow-up. *Rheumatology* 39: 894–902.

Gran JT, Skomsvoll JF (1997) The outcome of ankylosing spondylitis: a study of 100 patients. *British Journal of Rheumatology* **36**: 766–771.

Granfors K, Marker-Herman E, De Keyser P, Khan MA, Veys EM, Yu DT (2002) The cutting edge of spondyloarthropathy research in the millennium. *Arthritis and Rheumatism* **46**: 606–613.

Gratacos J, Collado A, Pons F and colleagues (1999) Significant loss of bone mass in patients with early, active ankylosing spondylitis: a followup study. *Arthritis and Rheumatism* **42**: 2319–2324.

Heikkila S, Viitanen JV, Kautiainen H, Kauppi M (2000) Sensitivity to change of mobility tests; effect of short term intensive physiotherapy and exercise on spinal, hip, and shoulder measurements in spondyloarthropathy. *Journal of Rheumatology* **27**: 1251–1256.

Herman M, Veys EM, Cuvelier C, De Vos M, Botelberghe L (1985) HLA-B27 related arthritis and bowel inflammation. Part 2: Ileocolonoscopy and bowel histology in patients with HLA-B27 related arthritis. *Journal of Rheumatology* **12**: 294–298.

Hidding A, van der Linden S, Gielen X and colleagues (1994) Continuation of group physical therapy is necessary in ankylosing spondylitis: results of a randomized controlled trial. *Arthritis Care Research* **7**: 90–6.

Holman H, Loric K (1987) Patient education in the rheumatic diseases: pros and cons. *Bulletin on the Rheumatic Diseases* **37**(5): 1–8.

Kahn M-F, Khan MA (1994) SAPHO syndrome. *Ballière's Clinical Rheumatology* **8**: 333–362.

Khan MA (1992) Spondyloarthropathies. *Rheumatic Disease Clinics of North America* **18**: 1–276.

Khan MA (1995) HLA-B27 and its subtypes in world populations. *Current Opinion in Rheumatology* **7**: 263–269.

Khan MA (1998) Slow-acting anti-rheumatic drugs in severe ankylosing spondylitis [Editorial]. *Journal of Clinical Rheumatology* **4**: 109–111.

Khan MA (2000) Patient-doctor. *Annals of Internal Medicine* **133**: 233–235.

Khan MA (2001) My self-portrait. *Clinical Rheumatology* **20**: 1–2.

Khan MA, Khan MK (1982) Diagnostic value of HLA-B27 testing in ankylosing spondylitis and Reiter s syndrome. *Annals of Internal Medicine* **96**: 70–76.

Khan MA, van der Linden SM (1990) A wider spectrum of spondyloarthropathies. *Seminars on Arthritis and Rheumatism* **20**: 107–113.

Khan MA, Khan MK, Kushner I (1981) Survival among patients with ankylosing spondylitis: a life-table analysis. *Journal of Rheumatology* **8**: 86–90.

Kidd BL, Cawley MI (1988) *Delay in diagnosis of spondarthritis*. British Journal of Rheumatology **27**: 230–232.

Koh TC (1982) Tai Chi and ankylosing spondylitis – A personal experience. *American Journal of Chinese Medicine* **10**: 59–61

Kraag G, Stokes B, Groh J, Helewa A, Goldsmith C (1990) The effects of comprehensive home physiotherapy and supervision on patients with ankylosing spondylitis: a randomized controlled trial. *Journal of Rheumatology* **17**: 228–233.

Laiho K, Tiitinen S, Kaarela K, Helin H, Isomaki H (1999) Secondary amyloidosis has decreased in patients with inflammatory joint disease in Finland. *Clinical Rheumatology* **18**: 122–123.

Lau CS, Burgos-Vargas R, Louthreno W, Mok MY, Wordsworth P, Zeng QY (1998) Features of spondyloarthritis around the world. *Rheumatic Disease Clinics of North America* **24**: 753–770.

Lloyd ME, Carr M, Mcelhatton P, Hall GM, Hughes RA (1999) The effects of methotrexate on pregnancy, fertility and lactation. *Quarterly Journal of Medicine* **92**: 551–563.

Lorig KR, Mazonson PD, Holman HR (1993) Evidence suggesting that health education for self-management in patients with chronic arthritis has sustained health benefits while reducing healthcare costs. *Arthritis and Rheumatism* **36**: 439–446.

McGonagle D, Khan MA, Marzo-Ortega H, O'Connor P, Gibbon W, Emery P (1999) Enthesitis in spondyloarthropathy. *Current Opinion in Rheumatology* **11**: 244–250.

Minden K, Kiessling U, Listing J, Niewerth M, Doring E, Meincke J, Schontube M, Zink A (2000) Prognosis of patients with juvenile chronic arthritis and juvenile spondyloarthropathy. *Journal of Rheumatology* **27**: 2256–2263.

NIH (1998) NIH Consensus Development Panel on Acupuncture. *Journal of the American Medical Association* **280**: 1518–1524.

Ostensen M, Ostensen H (1998) Ankylosing spondylitis – the female aspect. *Journal of Rheumatology* **25**: 120–124.

Pal B (1998) What counseling do patients with ankylosing spondylitis receive? Results of a questionnaire survey. *Clinical Rheumatology* **17**: 306–308.

Pato E, Banares A, Jover JA and colleagues. (2000) Undiagnosed spondyloarthropathy in patients presenting with anterior uveitis. *Journal of Rheumatology* **27**: 2198–2202.

Prieur AM (1998) Spondyloarthropathies in childhood. *Baillière's Clinical Rheumatology* **12**(2): 287–307.

Reveille JD, Ball EJ, Khan MA (2001) HLA-B27 and genetic predisposing factors in spondyloarthropathies. *Current Opinion in Rheumatology* **13**: 265–72.

Roldan CA, Chavez J, Wiest PW, Qualls CR, Crawford MH (1998) Aortic root disease and valve disease associated with ankylosing spondylitis. *Journal of the American College of Cardiology* **32**: 1397–1404.

Rosenberg AM (2000) Juvenile onset spondylo-arthropathies. *Current Opinion in Rheumatology* **12**: 425–429.

Santos H, Brophy S, Calin A (1998) Exercise in ankylosing spondylitis: How much is optimum? *Journal of Rheumatology* **25**: 215–60.

Sochart DH, Porter ML (1997) Long-term results of total hip replacement in young patients who had ankylosing spondylitis. Eighteen to thirty-year results with survivorship analysis. *Journal of Bone and Joint Surgery (America)* **79**: 1181–1189.

Strobel ES, Fritschka E (1998) Renal diseases in ankylosing spondylitis: review of the literature illustrated by case reports. *Clinical Rheumatology* **17**: 524–530.

Suarez-Almazor ME, Kendall CJ, Dorgan M (2001) Surfing the net—Information on the World Wide Web for persons with arthritis: Patient empowerment or patient deceit? *Journal of Rheumatology* **28**: 185–191.

Tico N, Ramon S, Garcia-Ortun F, Ramirez L, Castello T, Garcia-Fernandez L, Lience E (1998) Traumatic spinal cord injury complicating ankylosing spondylitis. *Spinal Cord* **36**: 349–352.

Uhrin Z, Kuzis S, Ward MM (2000) Exercise and changes in health status in patients with ankylosing spondylitis. *Archives of Internal Medicine* **160**: 2969–2975.

van der Heijde D, Calin A, Dougados M, Khan MA, van der Linden S, Bellamy N (1999) Selection of instruments in the core set for DC-ART, SMARD, physical therapy, and clinical record keeping in ankylosing spondylitis. Progress report of the ASAS Working Group. Assessments in Ankylosing Spondylitis. *Journal of Rheumatology* **26**: 951–954.

van der Linden SM *et al.* (1984) The revised New York criteria for ankylosing spondylitis. *Arthritis and Rheumatism* **27**: 361–368.

van der Linden SM, Valkenberg HA, de Jongh B, Cats A (1984) The risk of developing ankylosing spondylitis in HLA-B27 positive individuals. A comparison of relatives of spondylitis patients with the general population. *Arthritis and rheumatism* **27: 241–249.**

van Royen BJ, De Gast A (1999) Lumbar osteotomy for correction of thoracolumbar kyphotic deformity in ankylosing spondylitis. A structured review of three methods of treatment. *Annals of Rheumatic Diseases* **58**: 399–406.

Ward MM (1999) Health related quality of life in ankylosing spondylitis. A survey of 175 patients. *Arthritis Care Research* **12**: 247–255.

White M, Dorman SM (2001) Receiving social support on line: implications for health education. *Health Education Research* **16**: 693–707.

Yagan R, Khan MA (1983) Confusion of roentgenographic differential diagnosis between ankylosing hyperostosis (Forestier's disease) and ankylosing spondylitis. *Clinical Rheumatology* **2**: 285–292.

Zeidler H, Mau W, Khan MA (1992) Undifferentiated spondyloarthropathies. *Rheumatic Disease Clinics of North America* **18**: 187–202.

Books and monographs

Calin A, Taurog JD (eds) (1998) *The spondylarthritides.* Oxford University Press, Oxford.

Khan MA (1990) Ankylosing spondylitis and related spondyloarthropathies. In: *Spine: State of the art reviews.* Hanley & Belfus, Philadelphia, PA.

Khan MA (1996) Ankylosing spondylitis: Clinical features. In: Klippel JH, Dieppe PA (eds) *Rheumatology,* 2nd edition. Mosby, London, p. 6.

Khan MA (1996) Back and neck pain. In: Bone RC (ed) *Current practice of medicine*. Churchill Livingstone, Edinburgh, pp. 1–14.

Khan MA (1998) Spondyloarthropathies. In: Hunder G (Ed). *Atlas of rheumatology*. Current Science, Philadelphia, pp. 5.1–5.24.

Lopez-Larrea C (ed) (1997) *HLA-B27 in the development of spondyloarthropathies*. RG Landes Company, Austin, TX.

van der Linden S (1997) Ankylosing spondylitis. In: Kelly WN, Harris ED, Ruddy S, Sledge CB (eds) *Textbook of rheumatology*, vol 2, WB Saunders, Philadelphia, pp. 969–982.

WHO (1980) International Classification of Impairment, Disabilities, and Handicaps. World Health Organization, Geneva.

Index

Achilles tendonitis   22, 103
  reactive arthritis 131
Actonel   67
Actron   40
acupuncture   54–6
addresses   145–9
Advil   40
aerobic exercises   81
age of onset
  AS   1, 20
  psoriatic arthritis 134
alcohol   37
alendronate   67
Aleve   40
alternative therapy, see
  nontraditional therapy
American Football   81
American Heart Association
  62
American Psychiatric
  Association   86
amitriptyline   40
amoxicillin   62
ampicillin   62
amyloidosis of the kidneys   70
Anaprox   39, 40
anesthesia   63–4
ankylosing hyperostosis   99
Ankylosing Spondylitis
  Association of British
  Columbia (ASABC)   145
Ankylosing Spondylitis
  Association of Ireland
  (ASAI)   147
Ankylosing Spondylitis Caring
  Society of R.O.C.   149
Ankylosing Spondylitis Group
  of New South Wales   145
Ankylosing Spondylitis Group
  of Queensland   145

Ankylosing Spondylitis Group
  of Western Australia   145
Ankylosing Spondylitis
  International Federation
  (ASIF)   82, 143
annulus fibrosus   104
Ansaid   39
antibiotics   140
antigen-presenting cells   122
antinuclear antibodies   97
anti-TNF therapy   4, 12,
  47–8, 88
  side-effects, possible   48–9
  sponydloarthropathies
    138–9
aortic valve incompetence
  108
apical fibrosis   109
apophyseal joints   104
archery   80
aromatherapy   57
arthroplasty (joint replacement)
  61, 79, 89
  prophylaxis   62
Arthrotec   39
Associação Nacional da
  Espondilite Anquilosante
  (ANEA)   147
Associazione Italiana
  Spondiloartrite Anchilosante
  (A.I.Sp.A)   147
atlantoaxial joint, spontaneous
  subluxation of the   69
Australia   145
Austria   145
autosomes   114
Axid   41
Ayurveda   57
azathioprine   140
Azulfidine   43

back pain
  causes other than AS   98–9
  course of AS   19
  early diagnosis of AS   14–16
badminton   80
balls, Swiss exercise   24
bamboo spine   19, 105
basketball   80–1
baths
  before exercise   24
  radon   50
Bechterew, Vladimir von   7
Bechterewreumatikernas
  Intresseorganisation (BERI)
  148
bee venom   57
Belgium   145
Bextra   39, 42
bicycling, stationary   25
bio-feedback   56
biologic response modifiers
  (biologicals)   48–9
bisphosphonates   67
body contact sports   81
bony ankylosis of the spine
  104, 105
bowling   81
boxing   81
braces   77, 87
breast-feeding   42, 43, 45, 79
burning out of   AS 4
bursae   106
bursitis   106
Butazolidin   40

calcitonin   67
calcium supplements   67
Campylobacter infection   128
Canada   145–6
cancer of pelvis and spine   99
car driving   81–2, 89
case history, typical   71–3
Cataflam   39

cauda equina syndrome   69–70
causes of AS   2, 111, 113
  see also HLA-B27
CD4+ T cells   123
CD8+ T cells   113, 122
cefazolin   62
Celebrex   39, 42
celecoxib   39, 42, 43
cervical spine   9
cervicitis   131
chest pain   105
childbirth   79, 87
children
  course of AS   3, 21–2
  limb joints, involvement of   1
  spondyloarthropathies   135–7
    undifferentiated   137–8
chiropractice 52, 89
Chlamydia infection   128,
  129, 140
choline magnesium trisalicylate
  39
chondroitin sulfate supplements
  53
chronic inflammatory bowel
  disease (IBD)   2, 14, 108,
  112
  treatment   141
cimetidine   41
circinate balanitis   132
clindamycin 62
Clinoril   39
Clostridium infection   128
colitis, ulcerative   2, 14, 108,
  126
  enteropathic arthritis   135
complementary therapy *see*
  nonstandard therapy
computed tomography (CT)
  96
conjunctivitis   130, 135
Conner, Bernard   7, 8
contact sports   81
Coordinadora Nacional de
  Espondilitis anquilosante
  148
copper bracelets   57
corsets   87

corticosteroids 88
  effectiveness 45–6
  iritis 107–8
  spondyloarthropathies 138,
    141
  psoriatic arthritis 139
cortisone 88
course of AS 3–4, 13–14,
  19–20, 132–3
  children 21–2
  gender differences 20–1
  older people 21
COX1 42
COX2 42–3
COX-2 specific NSAIDs
  42–3
C-reactive protein (CRP)
  97
  case history 72
Croatia 146
Crohn's disease 2, 14, 108,
  112, 126
  enteropathic arthritis 135
  treatment 141
cross-country skiing 80
cycling
  long-distance 81
  stationary 81, 139
cyclo-oxygenase (COX)
  42–3
cyclosporin 139
cytokines 46
cytotoxic T cells 113, 122
Czech Republic 146

Daypro 39
Denmark 146
depression 85–6
Deutsche Vereinigung Morbus
  Bechterew (DVMB) 146
developing countries
  juvenile AS 21
  limb joints, involvement of 1
  spondyloarthropathies 128
diagnosis 1

back pain, other causes of
  98–9
  early 14–17
  HLA-B27 testing 117–18
  laboratory findings 97–8
  New York criteria 98
  radiology 95–6
  reactive arthritis 132
diclofenac 39
diclofenac sodium plus
  misoprostol 39
diets 37, 53, 87
diffuse idiopathic skeletal
  hyperostosis (DISH) 99
diflunisal 39
dimethyl sulfoxide (DMSO)
  57
disalcid 39
disease-modifying
  anti-rheumatic drugs
  (DMARDs) 43
DISH 99
diving, avoidance of 25
DMSO (dimethyl sulfoxide)
  57
Dolobid 39
dowager's hump 66
downhill skiing 81
driving 81–2, 89
drug therapy 37–8,
  87–8
  effectiveness 38
    corticosteroids 45–6
    COX-2 specific NSAIDs
      42–3
    methotrexate 44–5
    NSAIDs 38–43
    sulfasalazine 43–4
  new treatments 49–50
    TNF-based therapy
      46–9
  osteoporosis 67
  storage of medications 50
  see also named drugs
Društvo za ankilozirajoči
  spondilitis Slovenije (DASS)
  148
dynamic posture 77

early symptoms   13–14
  diagnostic pointers   14–17
earning capacity, AS's impact on
  82–4
Elavil   40
elderly people, course of AS
  21
elimination diets   53
employment, AS's impact on
  82–4
Enbrel   48
enteropathic arthritis   137
enthesitis   22, 103–5
  early detection   96
  spondyloarthropathies
    childhood   136, 139
    psoriatic arthritis   134
    reactive arthritis   131
    undifferentiated   137
enthesopathy, *see* enthesitis
epidural anesthesia   63
erythrocyte sedimentation rate
  (ESR)   97
  case history   72
  reactive arthritis   132
erythromycin   62
esomeprazole   41
Estratab   67
estrogen   67
etanercept   48
ethnicity, *see* race and ethnicity
etodolac   39
European Spondyloarthropathy
  Study Group (ESSG)   126,
  127
Evista   67
Excedrin   40
exercise and physical therapy
  23–5, 88–9
  heat, application of   25–6
  muscle-strengthening and
    stretching exercises   28–36
  posture   77, 78–9
  rheumatologist's role   92–3
  spinal extension and deep
    breathing exercises   26–7
  spondyloarthropathies   139

swimming   25
  see also sports
eye inflammation   2, 4, 14,
  107–8
  course of AS   20

facet joints   104
facts about AS   1–4
falls, avoiding   25, 75
family history   2, 10–12
  see also genetics
family life   79–80
family studies, HLA-B27
  123–4
famotidine   41
Feldene   39
fenoprofen   39
fertility   79, 87
fiber optic laryngoscopes   63
fibromyalgia   16, 21
fibrosis, apical   109
fibrositis   16, 21
Flanders   145
flurbiprofen   39
Food and Drug Administration
  (FDA), US   51
Forestier's disease   99
Fosamax   67

gadolinium 96
genetic counseling   115–17
genetics   2, 10–12, 111–12
  psoriatic arthritis   134
  see also HLA-B27, genetics
Germany   146
girdle joints   14, 105
  see also hip
glomerulonephritis   70
glucosamine supplements
  53
gluteal tuberosity   10
golfing   81
Great Britain   146
guided imagery   56

H2–blockers   41
health-related quality of life
   84–6
heart block   108
heart complications   62–3, 84,
   89, 108
heat, application of   25–6,
   139
heel pain   4, 22, 102–3
   reactive arthritis   131–3
helper T cells   123
herbal therapies   54
hiking   80
hip   105
   arthroplasty   61, 79, 89
   fracture   66
history, AS in 7
HLA (human leucocyte
   antigens)   112–13, 122–3
HLA-B27   2, 111–13
   genetics   10–12, 114–15
      counseling   115–17
      family studies   123–4
   research   122–3
      association with AS   122
      family studies   123–4
      prevalence in world population
         118, 119–21
   types   118, 120
   role in disease predisposition
      113–14
   spondyloarthropathies   125
      childhood   136, 137
      psoriatic arthritis   135
      reactive arthritis   126, 128,
         129, 133
   testing in disease diagnosis
      117–18
hockey 81
holistic medicine   56
homeopathy   53
Hrvatsko društvo za
   ankilozantni spondilitis
   146
human leucocyte antigens
   (HLA)   112–13, 122
   see also HLA-B27

Hungary   146
hydrotherapy   24, 89
hypnosis   56

ibuprofen   39, 40
IgA kidney disease   70
ilium   10
imagery, guided   56
Imuran   140
Indocid   39
Indocin   39
indomethacin   39, 42
infections as triggers
   AS   111
   reactive arthritis   126, 128,
      129
inflammatory bowel disease
   (IBD)   2, 14, 108, 112
   treatment   141
infliximab   48, 141
inheritance, *see* genetics;
   HLA-B27, genetics
interdisciplinary co-operation
   92–3
international AS organization
   143
Internet   59, 86, 144–50
Ireland   147
iritis, acute   2, 4, 14, 107–8
   course of AS   20
   psoriatic arthritis   130
   reactive arthritis   130
Italy   147

Japan   147
Japan Ankylosing Spondylitis
   Club   147
jaw   106
joint replacement (arthroplasty)
   61
   prophylaxis   62
juvenile AS   21–2
juvenile spondyloarthropathies
   135–7

keratinocytes   133
keratoderma blennorrhagica
    131
ketoprofen   39, 40, 43
ketorolac tromethamnine   39
kidney dysfunction   70
Klebsiella bacteria   111
Klub bechtěreviků   146
knee   21, 22, 136
Krebs, Hans Adolf   7
kyphosis   62

laboratory findings   97–8
    case history   72
Landsforeningen af Morbus
    Bechterew Patienter   146
lansoprazole   41
laryngoscopes, fiber optic   63
later manifestations of AS   70
    neurological problems   69–70
    osteoporosis   65–7
    spinal fracture   67–9
leukemia   138
limb joints, involvement of
    14, 105–6
literature, AS in   7
living with AS   3
    car driving   81–2
    depression   85–6
    employment and earning
        capacity, AS's impact on
        82–4
    falls, avoiding   75
    family life   79–80
    posture   75–7
        dynamic   77
        occupational   77–9
    quality of life, health-related
        84–5
    sports and recreational
        activities   80–1
local AS organizations
    143–49
Lodine   39

low-starch diets   53
lumbar spine   9
lung complications   63, 84,
    108–9
lung function testing   109

magnetic resonance imaging
    (MRI)   96
    undifferentiated
        spondyloarthropathy   138
magnets   57
management of AS, *see*
    treatment
Manitoba Ankylosing
    Spondylitis Association   145
Marie, Pierre   7
massage   52, 89
meclofenamate   39
Meclomen   39
meditation   54
MEDLINE Plus   59
mefenamic acid   39
meloxicam   39
men, course of   AS 20
methotrexate
    effectiveness   44–5
    spondyloarthropathies   138,
        139, 140–1
methyl sulfonyl methane
    (MSM)   57
Miacalcin   67
Mobic   39
Motrin   39, 40
Mozgáskorlátozottak
    Egyesületeinek Országos
    Szövetsége, Bechterew section
    148
muscle-strengthening and
    stretching exercises   28–36
myths about AS   3–4

nabumetone   39
Nalfon   39

naloxone   55
Naprelan   39
Naprosyn   39
naproxen   39, 40
naproxen sodium   39
national ankylosing spondylitis
   organizations   143–9
National Ankylosing
   Spondylitis Society (NASS)
   146
National Center for
   Complementary and
   Alternative Medicine
   (NCCAM) 58
National Institute of Mental
   Health   86
National Institutes of Health
   (NIH)   59
nature of AS   5–6
   developments in treatment
      12
   family history   10–12
   history, AS in   7
   literature, AS in   7
   sacroiliac joint   10
   spine, structure of   9–10
   terminology   7–8
Nederlandse bond van
   verenigingen van patiënten
   met reumatische
   aandoeningen, Commissie
   Morbus Bechterew   147
Netherlands   147
neurological problems
   69–70
New York criteria   98
Nexium   41
nimesulide   39
nizatidine   41
non-spinal (limb) joints,
   involvement of   105–6
non-steroidal anti-inflammatory
   drugs (NSAIDs)   12,
   87–8
   COX-2 specific   42–3
   effectiveness   38–43
   spondyloarthropathies   138
      unresponsive to   *140–1*

nontraditional therapy   51–2,
   56–8
   diets   53
   finding out about   58–9
   homeopathy   53
   Internet   59
   traditional Chinese medicine
      54–6
Norsk Revmatikerforbund
   (NRF)/Bekhterev   147
North American Spondylitis
   Consortium (NASC)
   149
Norway   147
NSAIDs, *see* non-steroidal
   anti-inflammatory drugs
Nuprin   40
nutritional supplements   53

occupational posture   77–9
oestrogen   67
older people, course of AS
   21
omeprazole   41
onycholysis   133
Ontario Spondylitis Association
   (OSA)   145–6
organizations, AS
   international   143
   national and local   143–9
   research   149–50
Orudis   39, 40
Oruvail   39
Osgood–Schlatter's disease
   138
osteitis condensans ilii   99
osteomalacia   99
osteophytes   99
osteoporosis   21, 65–8
   back pain   99
   drug therapy   67
Österreichische Vereinigung
   Morbus Bechterew (ÖVMB)
   145
oxaprozin   39

Index

Pagets disease   99
pamidronate   49
paraplegia   89
pelvis, cancer of the   99
penicillin   62
Pepcid   41
peptides   112, 122–3
personalized information cards
   68–9
phenylbutazone   12, 39, 40
physical therapy, see exercise
   and physical therapy
pink eye   130
piroxicam   39
placebo effect, nontraditional
   therapy   52, 55
plantar fasciitis   22, 103
   reactive arthritis   134
Ponstel   39
Portugal   147
posture   19, 75–7, 88
   dynamic   77
   exercise and physical therapy
      23, 24
   occupational   77–9
pregnancy   79, 87
   drug therapy   42, 43, 45, 79
Premarin   67
Prempro   67
Prevacid   41
prevalence
   AS   3
   HLA-B27   118, 120, 122
   reactive arthritis   129
Prilosec   41
process of AS   101–2
   enthesitis   103–5
   eye inflammation   107–8
   non-spinal (limb) joints,
      involvement of   105–6
   other structures, involvement
      of   106, 108–9
progesterone   67
prophylaxis   62
prostatitis   131
proton pump inhibitors   41

psoralen-photo-augmented
   ultraviolet A (PUVA)
   treatment   139
psoriatic arthritis   2, 126, 132,
   133–5
   childhood   137
   treatment   139–40
pubic junction   10
pubis   10
PUVA treatment   139

quadriplegia   68
quality of life, health-related
   84–5

race and ethnicity
   HLA-B27   117, 118, 119–21
   osteoporosis   66
   psoriatic arthritis   134
   reactive arthritis   133
radiation therapy   49–50, 89
radiology   95–6
radium chloride   50
radon bath   50
radon gas inhalation   49–50
raloxifene   67
Ramses II   7
ranitidine   41
reactive arthritis (Reiter's
   syndrome)   2, 126–28
   causes   111
   children   137
   diagnosis   133
   outcome   132–3
   prevalence   129
   symptoms   130–2
   treatment   140
recreational activities   80–1
Reiter's syndrome, see reactive
   arthritis
Relafen   39
Remicade   48, 141
remission   4, 14

research 122–3
  HLA-B27
    association with AS 122
    family studies 123–4
    prevalence in world populations 118, 119–21
    types 118–21
  organizations 149–50
Reston, James 55
rheumatoid arthritis 21
rheumatoid factor 97
rheumatologist's role 91–2
  interdisciplinary co-operation 92–3
Rheumatrex 44, 138, 140
risedronate 67
rofecoxib 39, 42
Rufen 40
rugby 81

sacroiliac joint 10, 11
  X-rays 2
sacroiliitis 13
  diagnosis 16, 95–6
  enteropathic arthritis 135
  psoriatic arthritis 135
  reactive arthritis 133–4
  X-rays 2
sacrum 10
S-Adenosylmethionine (SAM-e) 53
Salazopyrin 43, 138
Salmonella infection 128, 129, 137
Salsalate 39
SAPHO syndrome 99
'sausage digits'
  psoriatic arthritis 134
  reactive arthritis 131
Scheuermann's disease 99
Schober test 16
Schweizerische Vereinigung Morbus Bechterew (SVMB) 148
sclerosis 104
SEA syndrome 136

selective estrogen receptor molecules (SERMs) 67
self-help groups 89
  see also organizations, AS
seronegative spondyloarthritis 97
sex chromosomes 114
Shigella infection 128, 137
shoulder 105
side-effects
  anti-TNF therapy 49, 88
  corticosteroids 45
  methotrexate 44–5
  NSAIDs 40–2, 43
  sulfasalazine 43, 44
Singapore 148
Singapore Ankylosing Spondylitis Club (SASC) 148
skiing 80, 81
skin lesions 131
sleep
  drug therapy 40
  posture 75–7, 88
Slovenia 148
slow-acting anti-rheumatic drugs 43, 44, 140–1
smoking 27, 37, 88
snake venom 57
snorkels 25
soccer 81
Society of Patients with Ankylosing Spondylitis (Bechterew's disease) 149
Spain 148
spinal extension and deep breathing exercises 26–7
spine
  bony ankylosis 104, 105
  cancer 99
  fracture 62, 65, 67–9, 84
    caused by chiropractice/massage 89
  mechanical deterioration 98–9
  radiation treatment 89
  structure 9–10
  surgery 62

splints 87
spondylitis
  psoriatic arthritis 135
  reactive arthritis 132–3
Spondylitis Association of
  America (SAA) 149
  Straight talk on spondylitis
    79–80, 82
spondyloarthropathies 22,
  125–6, 127
  childhood (juvenile)
    135–7
  enteropathic arthritis 135
  psoriatic arthritis 133–5,
    139–40
  reactive arthritis 126–33
  treatment 138–9
    methotrexate 140–1
    *of skin involvement in psoriatic
      arthritis 139–40*
    sulfasalazine 140–1
  undifferentiated 137–9
spondylodiscitis 69
spondylosis 5
spontaneous subluxation of the
  atlantoaxial joint 69
sports 23, 80–1
stationary cycling 81, 139
storage of medications 50
Straight talk on spondylitis
  79–80, 82
Strümpell, Adolf 7
sulfasalazine
  effectiveness 43–4
  spondyloarthropathies 138,
    139, 140–1
sulindac 39
support groups 89
  see also organizations, AS
surgical treatment 62–3,
  89
  anesthesia 63–4
  joint replacement
    (arthroplasty) 61
    prophylaxis 62
  spondyloarthropathies 139
Sweden 148
swimming 25, 80, 89

spondyloarthropathies 139
Swiss therapeutic exercise balls
  24
Switzerland 148
symptoms
  AS 1, 13–14
  spondyloarthropathies
    childhood 136–7
    enteropathic arthritis 135
    psoriatic arthritis 133–4
    reactive arthritis 130–21
    undifferentiated 137–8
syndesmophytes 104

Tagamet 41
Tai Chi 54
Taiwan 149
temporo-mandibular joint 106
tendinitis 106
tendons 106
tennis 80
tenoxicam 39
TENS 56
terminology 7–8
thalidomide 49
thoracic spine 9
tiaprofenic acid 39
tibial tubercle 22, 136
TNF 46–7
  anti-TNF therapy 4, 12,
    47–8, 88
    side-effects, possible 48–9
    sponydloarthropathies 138–9
Tolectin 39
tolmetin 39
Toradol 39
total hip arthroplasty (THA)
  61, 79, 89
tracheostomy 63
traditional Chinese medicine
  (TCM) 54–6
transcutaneous electrical nerve
  stimulation (TENS) 56
treatment 2, 4
  developments 12
  overview 87–9

spondyloarthropathies 138–9
  *skin involvement in psoriatic
    arthritis* 11–2
  methotrexate 140–1
  sulfasalazine 140–1
  see also drug therapy; exercise
    and physical therapy;
    nontraditional therapy;
    surgical treatment
Trisilate 39
tumor necrosis factor alpha, *see*
  TNF

Ukraine 149
ulcerative colitis 2, 14, 108,
  126
  enteropathic arthritis 135
undifferentiated
  spondyloarthropathy
  137–8
United Kingdom 146
United States of America
  149
urethritis 130–1
US Food and Drug
  Administration (FDA) 51

uveitis, anterior 107
valdecoxib 39, 42
Valentini 7
venom, bee and snake 57
Vioxx 39, 42

vitamin supplements 53
  vitamin D 139
Vlaamse Vereniging voor
  Bechterew-patiënten (VVB)
  145
volleyball 80–1
Voltaren 39
von Bechterew, Vladimir 7

walking 80
Web sites 59, 86, 144–9
Welty, Eudora 7
women
  course of AS 3, 20–1
  osteoporosis 65–6
  see also breast-feeding;
    pregnancy
World Health Organization
  (WHO) 55
World Wide Web 59, 86,
  144–9

X-rays 2, 16, 95–6

Yersinia infection 128, 137

Zantac 41